STOP Thumb Suck Revolution™

37 HABIT BUSTERS TO HELP YOU
OR YOUR CHILD STOP THUMB, FINGER,
TOE, BLANKET *and* PACIFIER SUCK

Donald Fox, DDS, MS

Warning:
A medical physical is always recommended before you start on any type of dental or medical treatment. If you have or think you have any medical condition that would not allow you to apply the techniques in this book, see your doctor. Ask your physician if you or your child is a candidate to use these techniques.

Stop Thumb Suck Revolution™: 37 Habit Busters to Help You or Your Child Stop Thumb, Finger, Toe, Blanket & Pacifier Suck
by Donald M. Fox
www.stopthumbsuckrevolution.com

First Printing – December 2017
ISBN: 978-1-68111-213-8

Published by:
Wasteland Press
www.wastelandpress.net

Disclaimer:
Any companies or celebrities in this book do not imply endorsement of these entities by *Dr. Fox or the publisher.* The book is sold *as is*, without warranty of any kind, either expressed or implied, respecting the contents of this book, including but not limited to implied warranties for the book's quality, performance, merchantability or fitness for any particular purpose. Due to the extreme number of variables in society that children and adults are exposed to and different mental capacities of each individual, no guarantees are given that any one person will stop a habit and this book is written to help one decide to stop with the ultimate decision comes from the individual themselves. The book is written to help an individual and/or their parents understand the habit better and to increase communication about the habit. Neither Dr. Donald Fox nor its dealers or distributors shall be liable to the purchaser nor any other person or entity with respect to any liability, loss or damage caused or alleged to have been caused directly or indirectly by the book.

CONTENTS

FOREWORD

The number of thumb suck Americans whether they are children or adults is estimated at 5 million, which indicates that current techniques have failed. It's not just the technique! It's the fact of *trying to stop a habit as thumb sucking* that also causes children and adults not to stop it.

That's why Dr. Fox's *Stop Thumb Suck Revolution* isn't your typical how to book. It was inspired from helping a child of a hygienist who came to get Dr. Fox's help in his first year of private practice.

While Dr. Fox tried to help her, he researched further and found no one had much success in the dental field to break this habit. In the mental field, not much was found except they felt children were shy and wanted to sit on the floor in the infantile position.

By the way, a hint into future chapters of this book is that nothing of this sort was found in a thumb sucker and the opposite was found. Most are bored, very smart and wait for a chance to create something in life if only given a chance and some guidance.

So, your new job is that of a "Thumb Suck Buster."

To confront one's thumb suck habit doesn't mean one can handle or control it, but Dr. Fox's *Stop Thumb Suck Revolution* will help you understand your new role to bust or stop this habit and to handle the thumb suck problem.

Read the book as an adventure. I not only see children, but adults who thumb suck stop and their personality change as if they were stuck back in time and finally realize they are living "now in the present" and no longer with this habit. Read the book as new data to learn, not just about thumb sucking.

> ***"Here I go again, another thumb suck trick. Why should I even try since I'll probably fail?"***

Few books address the problems of thumb suck from the viewpoint of the thumb sucker. Instead, they are presented to us in a cartoon book or from a quick thing they learned from a school nurse, teacher or friend at a soccer game along with very little usable data.

This isn't good enough! People today are too smart for this. They want more information so they can think and make decisions for themselves while helping to stop themselves or their child from this mental and physical damaging habit.

Parents want their children not to be in the public eye seen as a child who's weak or something is wrong with them as shyness or something else.

More importantly, all dentists know that a child who sucks their thumb past the age of four will damage their teeth and bone structures that won't be self-corrected just by getting the thumb out of the mouth one day.

Damage will need corrected at age six by an orthodontist formally trained in early treatment to not only move the teeth, but move the bone structures of the upper and lower jaws. The problem today is that too many family dentists and parents have an old school mentality to wait to correct crooked teeth until after all the permanent teeth have erupted.

The problem with this thought process is that, by age twelve, the bones will be too hard to correct the bone damage from the thumb suck habit. And, this usually requires jaw surgery in addition to the braces that could have been avoided.

The bones at age six are very soft and allow a trained orthodontist to reverse the damage the thumb suck caused. The damages caused and the treatment for each damage will be outlined later in this book.

This book was written for parents to help their children stop the thumb or finger suck habit fast with less stress never known before in history. There's even a chapter on handling children who use a pacifier or "binky" past age two that causes the same damage as thumb sucking.

I knew that I had to write a book that would make a major difference in a child's or adult's life, stop their habit and at the same time have them feel good about themselves.

Now, when someone asks, "How did you stop that child's thumb suck habit so fast?" I say, "All the power a child needs to stop their habit is within my book."

Donald M. Fox, D.D.S., M.S.
Diplomate of the American Board of Orthodontics

DR. DONALD FOX

Dr. Fox is a Diplomate of the American Board of Orthodontics. He graduated number one out of his dental class of 115 and has received numerous awards in Dentistry.

The American Association of Orthodontists recognized him with the Harry Sicher award for the most meritorious first research in the United States and Canada. Dr. Fox discovered birth defects in animal studies, from low dosages of aspirin or acetaminophen taken during pregnancy.

He's the only doctor in the world who has learned how to stop a child or adult thumb, finger, toe, blanket and pacifier suck habit within a week without any appliances.

Dr. Fox is a problem solver. He tackles problems presented to him in his practice and life. And, he loves to teach others simpler methods to improve their lives. He's involved in other research projects.

He maintains a private practice in Florida. He has contributed time and financial resources to the Clearwater Aquarium in Clearwater, Florida that rescues stranded and injured marine wildlife and helps them return to nature.

Dr. Fox cares about others and this has led him to write this book so that everyone will know and benefit from his secrets to stop the thumb, finger, toe, blanket and pacifier habits. Read more about Dr. Fox in "About the Author" in the last section of this book.

PREFACE

Let me tell you the story about the first thumb sucker who came to my office that helped me develop what's in this book. She was six years old and the daughter of a dental hygienist. The dental hygienist stated she was embarrassed by the fact that she didn't stop the child's thumb suck habit.

Interestingly, many parents have this same guilty feeling. She had tried numerous things to get her to stop. After I worked with the child numerous visits the child stopped and the mother came forward and stated I did an awesome job, but she was further embarrassed to tell me that her child also sucked her right large toe.

My first response was, of course, "Why didn't you tell me?" She stated, "I'm embarrassed and thought she would stop the toe habit when she stopped the thumb habit." I then asked, "Was there anything else that I need to know about? She said, "No." And, we all laughed.

We did the same techniques all over again and she stopped the toe suck. Then, the child told me ... and the mother didn't think anything about it ... that she also sucked a blanket. She took the corner of a small blanket and folded it up into a knot and sucked on it.

We then went through the technique a third time to get her off that. It was at that time we noticed the changes in her, as mentioned later in this book, about how a child doesn't seem like a baby any more and more importantly they no longer talk like one. Yes, many thumb suckers still not only suck as a one-year-old, but act and talk like one ... yet this magically disappears when the thumb habit vanishes.

To handle the problem, I dug into books and discovered things I really hadn't understood about thumb sucking. I found misleading facts I had been told in the past and assumed were true.

Once I cleared up the confusions on why children and adults thumb suck, I started to think the opposite of how everyone else did including psychologists. Then, the cure for thumb sucking was discovered. Children and adult thumb suckers didn't lack psychiatric chemicals in their brain that caused them to suck.

There are patients who exist who do have mental problems... let's get real. I don't want to argue with the mental field, but most thumb sucker patients don't fit into this scenario.

This thumb suck problem needs handled little by little in the proper sequence. One doesn't go to second grade without completing first grade.

This book is laid out so that you don't jump into the thumb suck habit cold turkey. It's designed to have you take baby steps and make permanent changes in the child or adult habit.

I've been a doctor for years and have helped over twenty thousand patients. When I focus my attention outward on my patients and others who need help, rewards come back to me in different forms many of which aren't noticed right away.

Back in fourth grade, I decided to dedicate my life to being a doctor to help people. That's the purpose why I wrote this thumb suck book for you!

CHAPTER 1

History of the Thumb Suck Habit

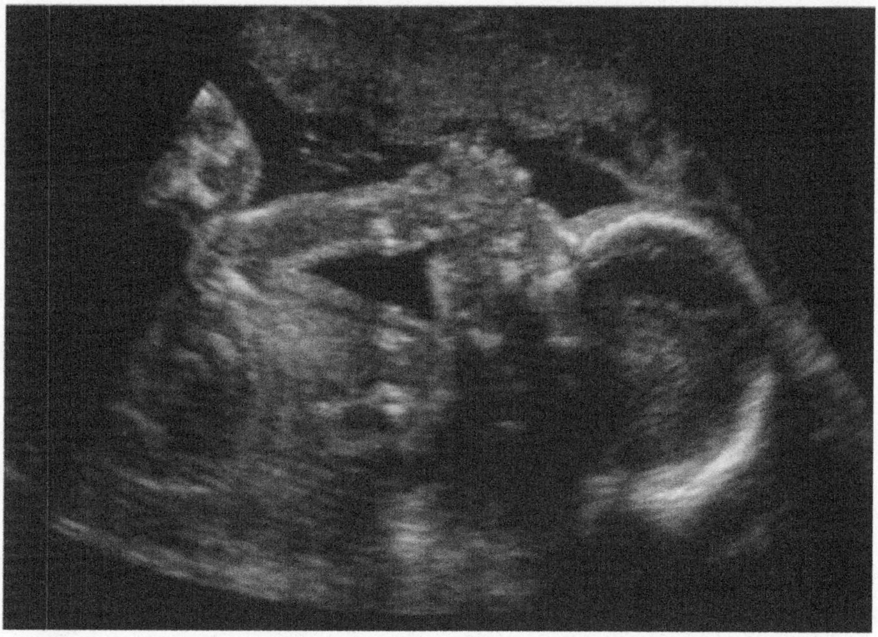

It's been known for years that the thumb suck habit can start as early as a fetus. Wikipedia in an article on thumb sucking stated that ultrasound scans have revealed the habit starts as early as fifteen weeks after the egg and sperm have joined in the womb. Others start as an infant between the ages of zero and one. I've had patients as old as thirty-one with the habit.

As far as when someone first wrote about how to stop the habit, the below is found in Wikipedia:

Hoffmann wrote *Struwwelpeter* in reaction to the lack of good children's books. He intended to buy a picture book as a Christmas present for his three-year-old son, Hoffmann instead wrote and illustrated his own book. In 1845, he was persuaded by friends to publish the book anonymously as:

> *Lustige Geschichten und drollige Bilder mit 15 schön kolorierten Tafeln für Kinder von 3–6 Jahren* (*Funny Stories and Whimsical Pictures with 15 Beautifully Coloured Panels for Children Aged 3 to 6*).

For the third edition, published in 1858, the title was changed to *Struwwelpeter*, the name of the character in the first story. The book became popular among children throughout Europe, and, writes author and researcher Penni Cotton, the pictures and characters showed a great deal of originality and directness.

Relationship between breast-fed & thumb suck

In 1977, researchers studied fifty children between ages one and seven who were habitual thumb suckers, and compared these with children who didn't suck their thumb. The studies showed that thumb suckers tended to be bottle-fed rather than breast-fed.

- The later the child was weaned (wean means to withdraw from something and in this case, means to withdraw a child from mother's milk breast-fed), the less likely he was to suck his thumb.
- The thumb suck children tended to have been fed on schedule rather than on cue.
- Ninety-six percent of the thumb suckers had been left to fall asleep alone after being fed. But, not one of the non-thumb suckers was left alone to fall asleep.

Therefore, researchers theorize that while asleep, persons return to primitive reflexes, such as "to suck and hand-to-mouth actions." In some pediatric practices, they noticed that babies who were nursed down to sleep and not weaned until they're ready were much less likely to become a habitual thumb sucker. They stated to consider breastfeed as a prevention of the thumb suck habit.

As Far as Devices Used in the Past
The Earliest Orthodontic Thumb Suck Device

In the Chicago Daily Tribune newspaper, Friday, September 12, 1952, an article appeared titled, *Dental Spurs Put the Bite on Thumb Sucking.* It claimed to be a device hitched to teeth called a cure by Northwestern University in Chicago. This was the first device perfected by Dr. Touro Graber, orthodontist.

It was a metal strip to which the spurs were attached ran across the roof of the mouth. Interestingly, he stated to parents not to worry about the habit unless it persisted beyond the child's third year. The article is seen below:

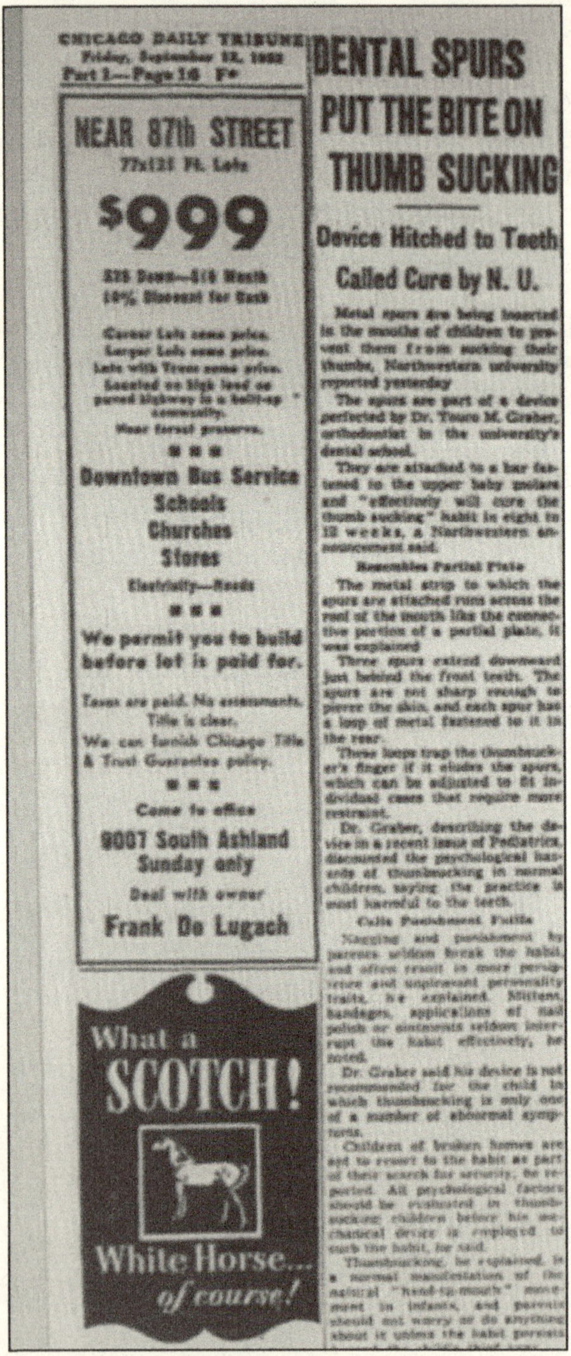

CHICAGO DAILY TRIBUNE
Friday, September 12, 1952
Part 1—Page 16 F*

NEAR 87th STREET
77x121 Ft. Lots
$999
$25 Down—$15 Month
10% Discount for Cash
Corner Lots same price.
Larger Lots same price.
Lots with Trees same price.
Located on high land on paved highway in a built-up community.
Near forest preserve.
Downtown Bus Service
Schools
Churches
Stores
Electricity—Roads
We permit you to build before lot is paid for.
Taxes are paid. No assessments. Title is clear.
We can furnish Chicago Title & Trust Guarantee policy.
Come to office
9007 South Ashland
Sunday only
Deal with owner
Frank De Lugach

What a SCOTCH!
White Horse... of course!

DENTAL SPURS PUT THE BITE ON THUMB SUCKING

Device Hitched to Teeth Called Cure by N. U.

Metal spurs are being inserted in the mouths of children to prevent them from sucking their thumbs, Northwestern university reported yesterday.

The spurs are part of a device perfected by Dr. Touro M. Graber, orthodontist in the university's dental school.

They are attached to a bar fastened to the upper baby molars and "effectively will cure the thumb sucking" habit in eight to 12 weeks, a Northwestern announcement said.

Resembles Partial Plate

The metal strip to which the spurs are attached runs across the roof of the mouth like the connective portion of a partial plate, it was explained.

Three spurs extend downward just behind the front teeth. The spurs are not sharp enough to pierce the skin, and each spur has a loop of metal fastened to it in the rear.

These loops trap the thumbsucker's finger if it eludes the spurs, which can be adjusted to fit individual cases that require more restraint.

Dr. Graber, describing the device in a recent issue of Pediatrics, discounted the psychological hazards of thumbsucking in normal children, saying the practice is most harmful to the teeth.

Calls Punishment Futile

Nagging and punishment by parents seldom break the habit, and often result in more persistence and unpleasant personality traits, he explained. Mittens, bandages, applications of nail polish or ointments seldom interrupt the habit effectively, he noted.

Dr. Graber said his device is not recommended for the child in which thumbsucking is only one of a number of abnormal symptoms.

Children of broken homes are apt to resort to the habit as part of their search for security, he reported. All psychological factors should be evaluated in thumbsucking children before his mechanical device is employed to curb the habit, he said.

Thumbsucking, he explained, is a normal manifestation of the natural "hand-to-mouth" movement in infants, and parents should not worry or do anything about it unless the habit persists

Thumb Guard:

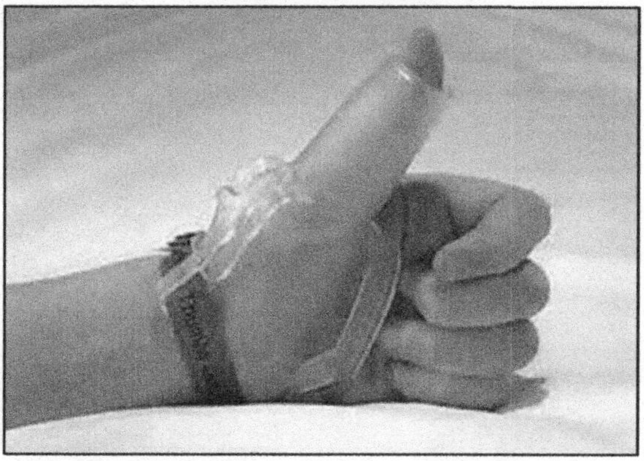

Two Finger Plastic Guard:

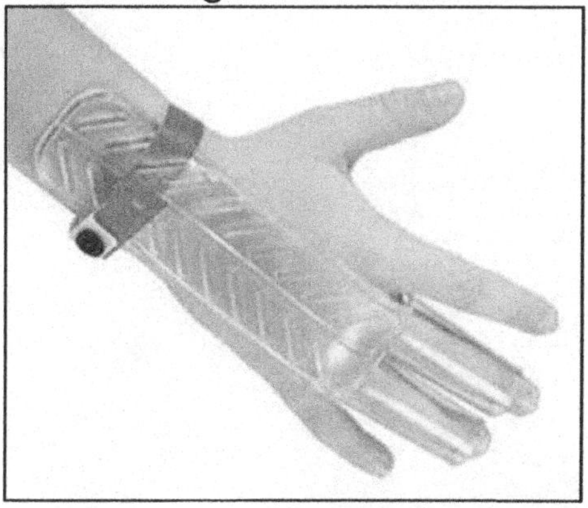

Middle Two Finger Glove:

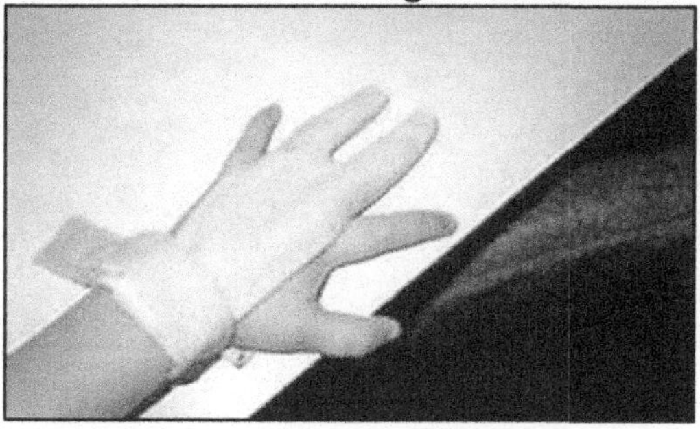

Thumb Glove:

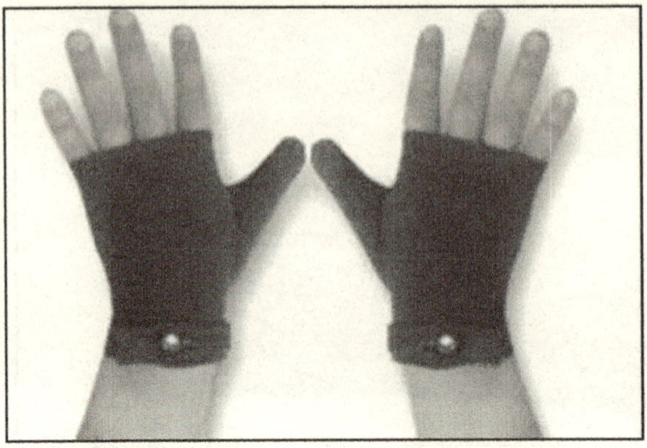

Crib Appliance Glued onto Teeth:

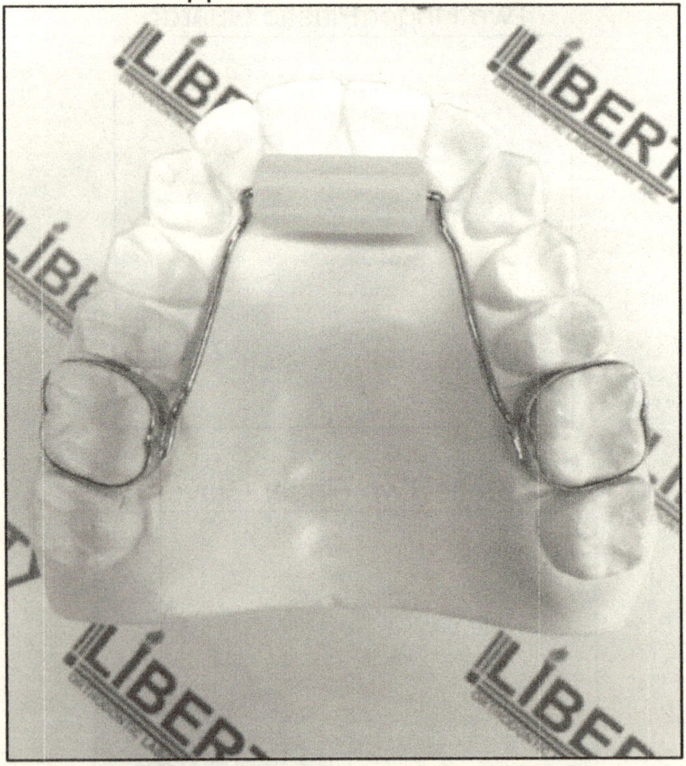

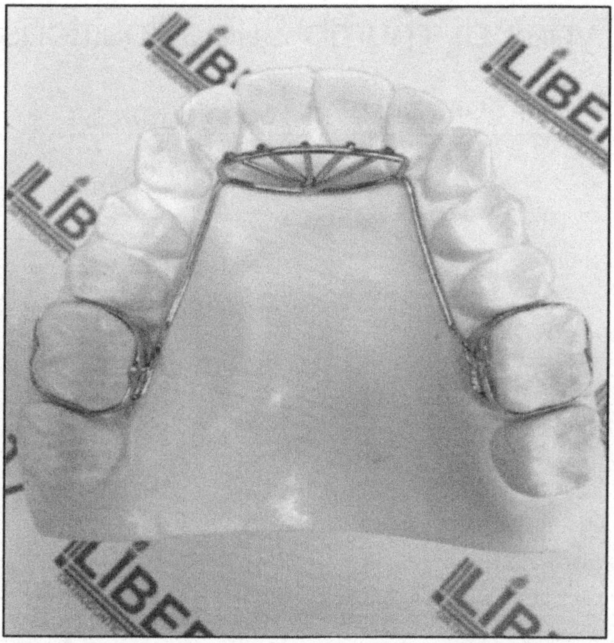

Crib Appliance with Reminder Spurs:

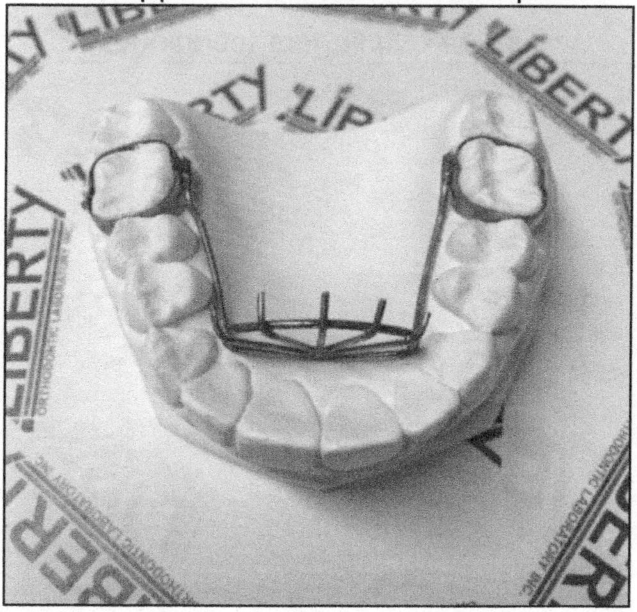

Types of Thumb Suck Positions

Whole Hand Technique:

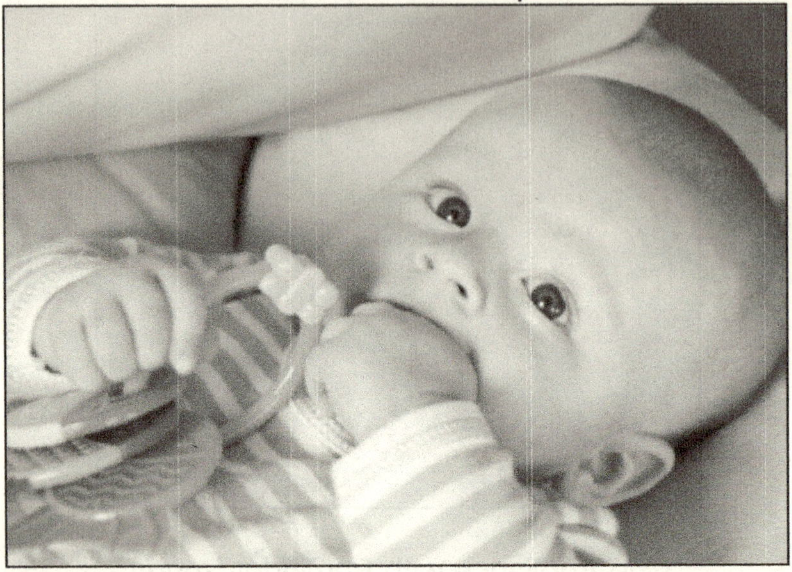

One or two fingers technique:

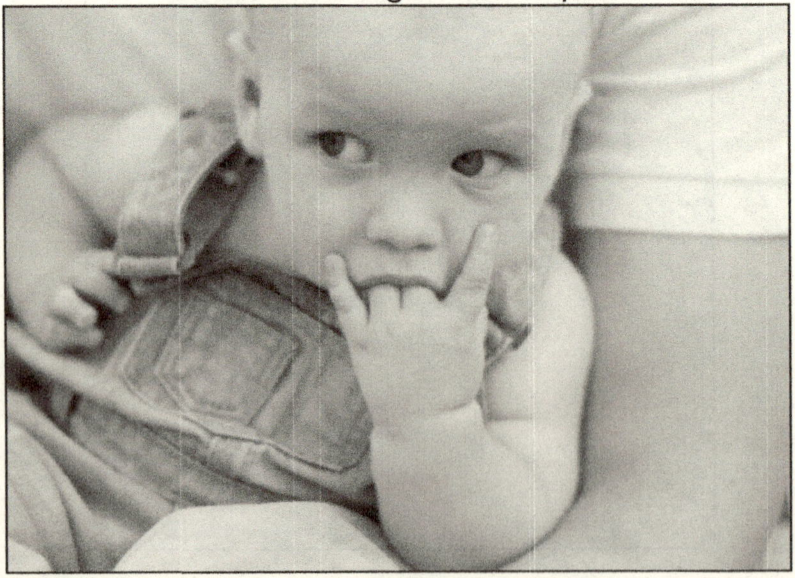

Thumb-nose technique:

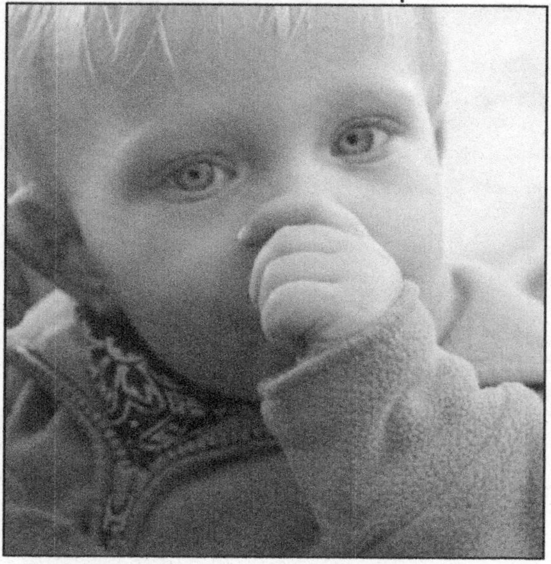

Upside down Thumb Technique:

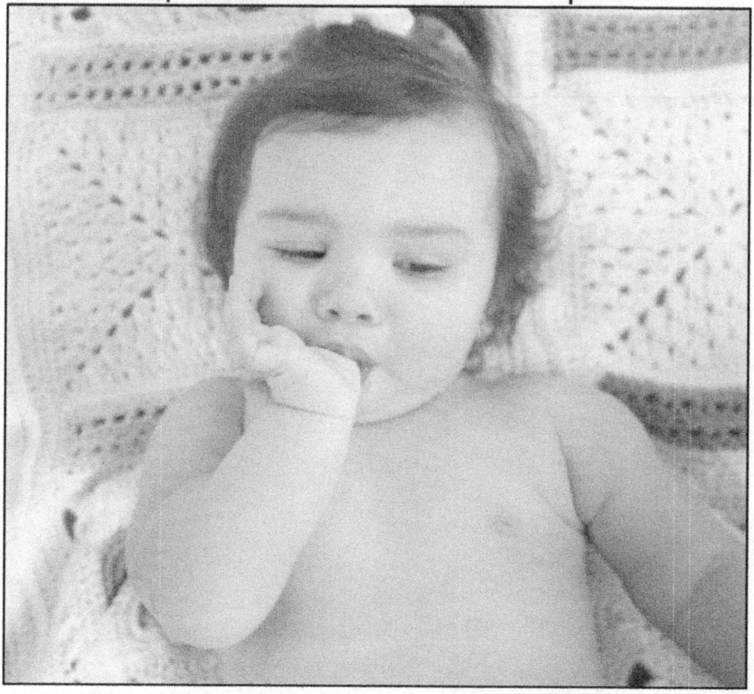

Old Fashion Technique:

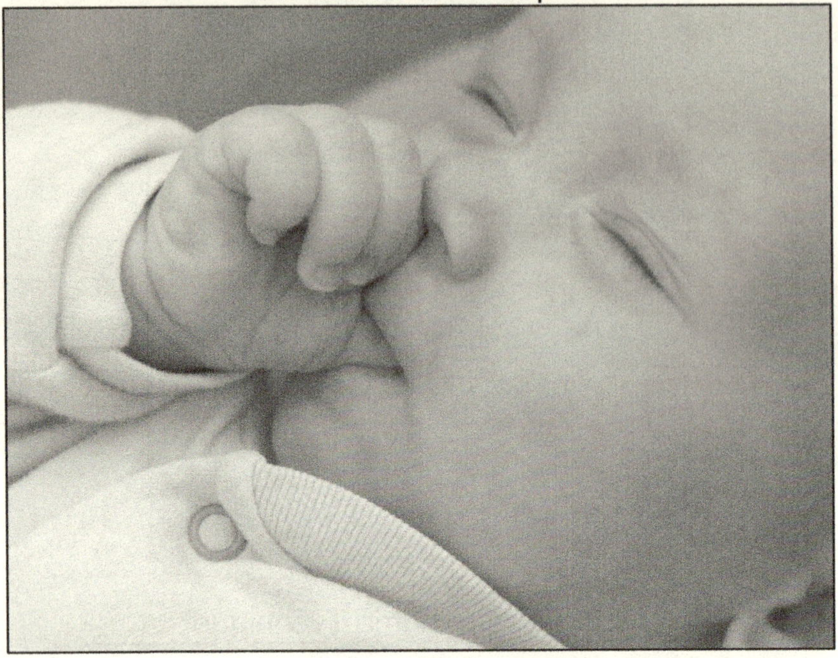

Toe Suck Technique:

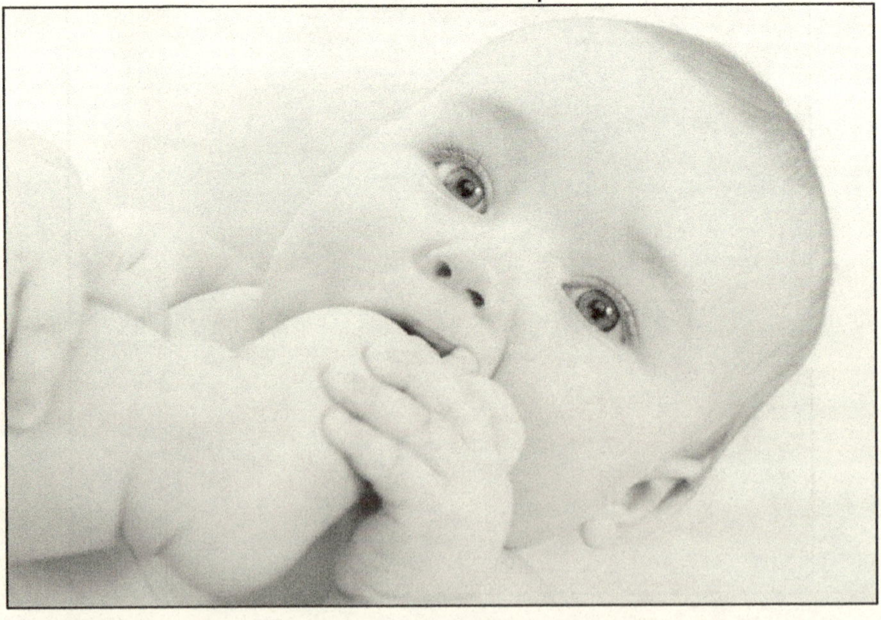

Binky or Pacifier Habit:

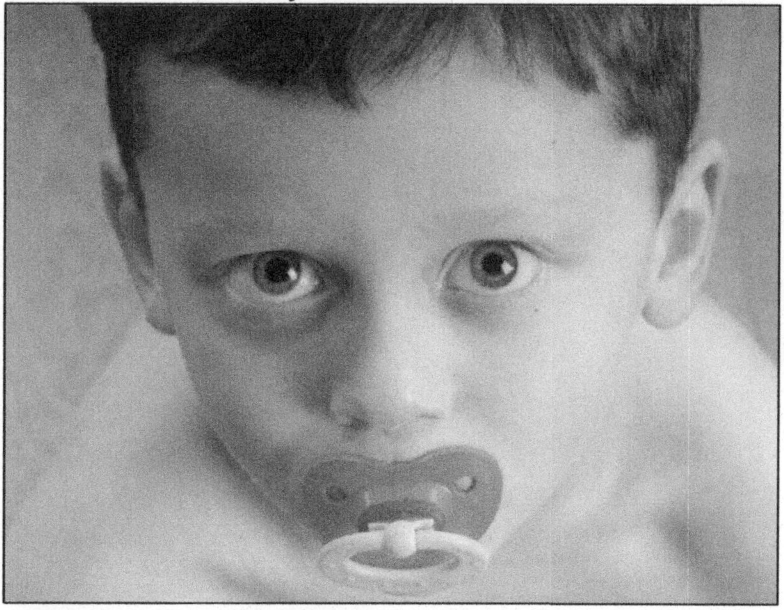

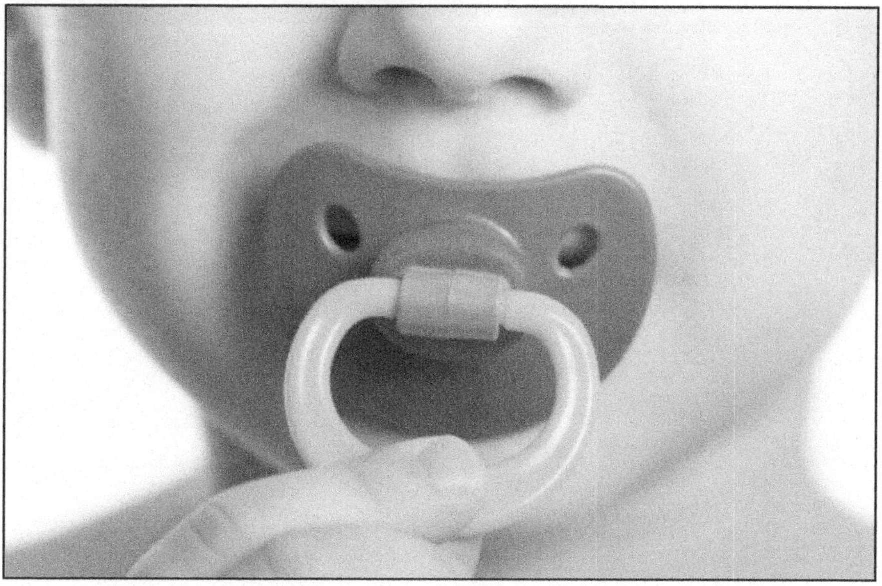

CHAPTER 2

False Information about Thumb Suckers

There's so much false information about thumb suckers:

- They're shy.
- They're introverted.
- They're the type that likely go hide in a closet in a fetal position and not confront life.
- For some reason, they need to suck and they must be allowed to suck.
- They'll grow out of their habit. Leave them alone.
- Kids suck their thumbs because it's comforting and calming.
- Your preschooler practiced this habit while she was still in the womb and perfected it as an infant.
- Now she turns to her thumb when she's tired, scared, bored, sick, or trying to adjust to challenges such as starting daycare or preschool.
- To help her fall asleep at bedtime and to lull herself back to sleep when she wakes up in the middle of the night.
- She indulges in the habit for comfort and security.

- The American Dental Association says most children can safely suck their thumb – without damaging the alignment of their teeth or jaws – until their permanent teeth begin to appear. (Permanent teeth don't usually start to erupt until around age 6.)

The worst one of all the false data above

Out of all the above, ***they'll grow out of their habit, leave them alone***, ranks as the worst false data. I just can't think with this one. Four reasons this is false:

1) First, that's totally contrary to recommendations by dentists and orthodontists worldwide and their associations, the American Dental Association and the American Association of Orthodontists. The damage to the teeth and bone structures starts between the ages of two and four years old will require age 6 early treatment orthodontic appliances done by a highly trained orthodontist in facial growth (Dentofacial Orthopedics).

   Amazingly, Wikipedia, under the topic of *Thumb Sucking*, states twice that it's been shown if the habit is broken before the onset of permanent teeth eruption into the mouth, at around five years old, the damage is reversible. This is false information since they quoted their information from an article in the Journal of Pediatrics, April 1994, titled, *"Influence of thumb sucking on pure social acceptance in first grade children."*

   I've found pediatric physicians aren't the experts in facial growth compared to orthodontists that have a degree in Dentofacial Orthopedics as I have. I see teeth and bone damage all the time in children that I treat at age six. They have jaw growth problems and sucked six years in a row. For that matter, when I see them for their first visit, I also see their younger age two or three brother or sister because they come together as a family. They also suck and have the same damage.

2) Second, speech problems will develop from the teeth and bone structures out of alignment. Especially if the child is allowed to develop their speech between the ages of two and six with the teeth and bones out of alignment.
3) Third, the older the thumb sucker is, the harder it is to deal with peer pressure. Also, they constantly feel fear to have to come out of the closet that someone at school or work will find out about their habit.
4) Fourth, the mannerism and speech immediate change from use of the techniques in this book demonstrate they have a ***less quality of life*** and they deserve the highest quality of life as an individual and human being.

Analogies to allow someone with a habit to grow out of it or magically disappear

- That's equivalent to allow a fourteen-year-old who's 100 pounds overweight to continue to overeat each day because they need to grow out of it.
- That's equivalent to allow a fourteen-year-old who smokes two packs of cigarettes a day because they need to grow out of it.
- That's equivalent to allow a fourteen-year-old who drinks a pint of bourbon daily because they need to grow out of it.

Introverted false data

I've seen in patients, I've cured of the thumb suck habit and expressed in more detail and other parts of this book, that they're the opposite of introverted. They're very creative, smart people and aren't introverted, but bored and don't create things in life.

Studies done on adult thumb suckers demonstrated they're affluent and well educated. There's no introversion found in this study.

I'll agree, if you go to a psychiatric hospital and find patients of any age who have serious mental problems whether they're medicated or not, that a thumb sucker will be found. But, to label thumb suckers generally as introverted personalities haven't been found to exist.

Even Shari Green, Certified in Orofacial Myology (disorders of the face, mouth, lips or jaw), stated in an article by Shannon Prather titled, "Thumb sucking is a hard habit to break," that, "The notions that thumb sucking is a symptom of a deep seated psychological problem are antiquated and simply wrong. In fact, many of her adult patients are educated and successful."

Questionable data theory

In a journal article, *Study of Oral Fixation: PICA,* in the Journal of the American Academy of Child and Adolescent Psychiatry, FK, Millican, et al., child psychiatrist, wrote the below:

"Pica is a depraved appetite with resultant ingestion of nonfood substances. Pica has been known since ancient times and found to occur on every continent (Anell and Lagercrantz, 1958; Cooper, 1957; Lau fer, 1930). In the United States at present, pica occurs most frequently among

the low-income Negro and white populations, and some Indian tribes; it is not so prevalent in the upper and middle income white population.

Children with pica had a high degree of other oral problems, including mouthing of objects, thumb sucking, and psychological feeding problems. They were somewhat retarded in speech development, and some withheld speech. They showed conflicts about their dependency needs and around handling of their aggressive feelings, and exhibited considerable negativism...

In those cases where economic or marital problems led to maternal deprivation, as a major causative factor in the child's pica, a casework approach was utilized. Many of the younger children were still sufficiently malleable in personality to benefit from this approach. If the child's psychopathology had developed to such an extent that these approaches were deemed insufficient, then psychotherapy was indicated."

So, in the above writing, they never did really figure out why children thumb suck and to relate children at a very young age who sucked on objects, finger or thumb being related to a mental disorder is questionable. Or, is it simply that this is what babies do or they're bored, hungry or something as simple as an adult who chews on a pen or chewing gum? Yes, I believe there's a child who has a severe mental issue who happens to then also put an object in their mouth or their thumb, but caution is given to the reverse to label children that do this with a mental issue.

False information about thumb sucking and the use of pacifiers

Nicholas Day, April 27, 2010, freelance writer in New Haven, Connecticut wrote many bullets of false information in an article titled, *Babies suck: The Twisted History of Pacifiers*:

- Pacifiers have been blamed from everything from masturbation to drug abuse. No wonder Nicholas day can't bear to let his son use one.
- In 1879 in a German medical journal, S. Lindnew, a German pediatrician, wrote that infantile sucking was the cause of chronic masturbation. Even though there were sixty-nine children in the study and only four of these followed in time masturbated he felt this was proof of his hypothesis.
- Freud, several decades later, wrote that infants who persist in the habit of sucking always become masturbators.
- Later, an English health pamphlet warned and so did a popular child care book of the time describe a pacifier user as feeble, nervous and timid. To take away the pacifier wasn't enough. Parents were instructed to tie their children's hands to their cribs and if that didn't work to out their hands inside aluminum mittens.
- In 1925 the American psychologist, James Mursell, went so far to argue that the smoking habit was caused by the urge to suck.
- By the early 1940s, while ideas emerged for the reason for thumb suck, there was no proof in a journal article by Joseph Gillman who observed thumb and toe suck in a baboon and two honey bears.

CHAPTER 3

How to Screen Children Who Not to Use This Book On

Certain children whom are difficult to work on are easily identified and mustn't apply the techniques in this book on. One child I remember never sat still in the chair and continued to get out of the chair and run around the room. I told mom that I'll try again in six months to see if the child matured.

I've had parents demand me to stop their child's thumb suck habit when I know it'll be an uphill battle with other factors that exist at home or in the child's life. I only accept patients who I know I can deliver a high percentage product on, so that the patient and their parents aren't the only ones happy with the result, but I'm happy, also.

I've successfully treated children as early as age two. Over one-third of age two children will sit still, talk back and forth as if they were an adult and keep eye contact with you. Those are the three minimal requirements.

The bone and the teeth start to get damaged at age two and the lower jaw is kept from forward growth if the thumb habit isn't stopped. I do have better success with children at six years old, but damage to the child's bone structures and teeth is prevented if stopped earlier.

Again, the point here is that communication is the key to the thumb sucker buster techniques to work. The best results are obtained on a child who'll have a discussion with you as if they were an adult and you can tell they're smart. After you first talk with the child and you don't feel that a back-and-forth discussion happened as if you had talked to your best friend, it's best not to push the situation because results won't be achieved or will take longer than usual.

If a child can't carry on an adult-like conversation and can't even answer a yes or no question, you'll need to wait another year before use of the techniques in this book, especially if the child is under five years old. I've worked with children as early as two, but they were very special and mature for their ages. These children started a conversation with me about a topic of their own.

Children on psychiatric drugs, as you can imagine, have a hard time with instructions much less follow through the steps in this book. The only failures I had were children on Ritalin who had attention deficit disorder (ADD or ADHD). It went nowhere after three attempts and I gave up. We eventually applied different other things as fixed appliances at a later age just to keep the thumb out of the mouth which is the way most Orthodontists and Pedodontists do it today. This doesn't get to the root of the problem which is the key point to this book – the child decides to stop without force or punishment. Appliances as these aren't usually welcomed by the child since they're a form of force and don't represent self-determinism.

Don't get me wrong or miscommunicate with me at this point, but this book is written for children who don't have many personal or family problems at home with their parents, don't receive psychological services or need psychiatric drugs. I don't have any research, testimonials or information about these types of patients and you're welcome to use the techniques in this book, but I don't support them.

The oldest patient that I've treated was a thirty-two-year-old woman. The youngest was one year and ten months. Surprisingly, most patients didn't arrive to me until the age of seven to nine years old which is too late.

I can't over-emphasize the need to stop the thumb suck habit no later than age four or five before the front teeth start to erupt. If possible, it's more advantageous to stop the habit at age two. There are other chapters devoted that explain the damage that occurs and how the damage is treated to avoid jaw surgery and braces at age sixteen.

CHAPTER 4

A Family Member Isn't the Best Person to Stop the Thumb Suck Habit

Most parents won't be able to apply these techniques in this book to their child. The child has already had negative events in the past with their parents. The child knows they're frustrated with them and can tell by certain words, actions and other types of cues the parents give. It's best to start with a clean slate.

The same's true about any family member. An adult thumb sucker's best friend, spouse or boyfriend/girlfriend isn't the best either.

It's been known for hundreds of years that many families don't have family members listen to each other even though they're supposed to because they're family members and there's some sort of family love there. Yet, every week, I hear stories of family problems where no one in the family listened or took family advice. It seems to be ingrained or implanted mentally that causes this to exist.

I've noticed this when "the family" tried to handle a teenage drinker or one who acted bad in school and the child already has put up their wall from the other family members.

No matter what the family may state: "They're here to help and won't be negative." It just won't work, sorry.

The parent must be present when these techniques are administered so there's nothing that comes across that makes the child feel bad or inferior. And, the parent does need to help at home after the techniques are applied and must be fully educated what to do.

To not have the parent present invites trouble of he-said-she-said miscommunication and the parent gets to hear "unusual" things from the child when they ask the child later, "What did you talk about today when they addressed your thumb suck habit?" This is whether it's with me or with someone else who applies these techniques.

It's best to get a neighbor who's super friendly that the child loves. The child must really admire this person. A good test of this is to have the child, asked by this neighbor, to go get the newspaper at the front door and the child brings it to them or to get a soda out of the refrigerator for the neighbor is a pretty good signal that they'll listen to this neighbor. Also, be sure the neighbor loves children and has patience to apply these techniques to your child.

The person selected needs to read this book to know all the techniques and not just apply parts of the book. When this friend or neighbor talks to the child they need to talk to them as an adult. It's appropriate that not only does the neighbor listen to the child, but acknowledges the child what they say to them and that the child be free to say whatever they want to and within reason. Acknowledge means to say to the child, I understand, or okay or repeat back to the child a shorter version what the child just said to the neighbor. This allows the child to realize they've been heard and that someone duplicates them.

Many families have brought children to me with poor communication about this problem done between all the family members. One or more parents yelled at the child or made them feel bad and the child had no chance to talk to the parent about the habit or the parent didn't want to listen. The key to the success of the thumb suck buster techniques is that the child is listened to, the child can feel duplicated about their problem and feel safe that someone really wants to help them.

CHAPTER 5

Preparation before the Start of the Thumb Suck Buster Techniques

Evaluation of the child's airway

Every child needs to breathe through their nose and mouth correctly. What's most important is the ability to breathe through the nose clearly. If a child has allergies, mouth breathes or has sleep apnea they'll have difficulty with the techniques in this book.

It's also advised that a child visit an ENT specialist (Ear, Nose and Throat) before use of these techniques if problems as these exist. I've personally seen clinically a correlation between children who have airway problems and children who suck their thumb or fingers. From a physiological standpoint, the airway works basically the same way a firehose does when it comes to resistance.

Resistance is observed with the diameter of the firehose and the pressure of the water that determines the flow of the water through the hose and out of the firehose strong enough to put out the fire. In the human body, resistance is seen with the diameter of the wind or air pipe to the lungs. If someone has airway problems, they'll adjust the diameter of their airway to the lungs with use of their finger or thumb in their mouth to increase the resistance to make the air flow in and out easier. Most of the time, the person with the airway problems doesn't realize they have figured out this solution to their problem, they only care that they can breathe easier.

This may explain the history of parents who state their child's more comfortable sucking their thumb and doesn't have anything to do with stress or introversion, but they found it easier to breathe with it in. In other locations of this book there are also things that contribute to the thumb suck habit other than airway problems as:

- The child's bored and very smart at the same time.
- The child's extroverted and feels trapped or stuck where they are in location and what they do at their age in life and feel they can't change it.
- The child has no creations or a low level of creations in life (discussed in detail later in this book).

If the adenoids and/or tonsils need removed than do so before the start of this book. A very well-trained orthodontist is trained in this area to diagnose the airway problems. There's an X-ray of the head called a Lateral Cephalogram (ceph) which means an X-ray taken from the side (lateral) of the head (ceph) that shows the entire skull and bones of the face and the airway that goes through the nose to the lungs and also the air from the mouth to the lungs that meet at the back of the throat.

A normal X-ray shows a half inch diameter of the airway "pipe" in the area of the adenoids located at the back of the nose. If the adenoids are large they'll cause the airway to decrease to zero or as small as one quarter of an inch to prevent air from the nose to the lungs.

For over twenty-five years, I've examined children for braces that I saw airway problems from across the room when I entered the room that the parents were totally blind to. To detect these in the thumb sucker you're about to help, you'll notice the mouth is usually open, have dark rings and puffiness under their eyes. Thumb suckers are often tired because they don't get into their deep Delta sleep and continue to wake up groggy into their rapid eye movement sleep.

The deep Delta sleep is needed to replenish the proteins of the body and the brain to feel fresh the next day. Rapid eye movement sleep (REM sleep, REMS) is a unique phase of sleep in mammals and birds, characterized by random movement of the eyes, low muscle tone throughout the body and the natural tendency of the sleeper to dream vividly.

The quality of life improvement with the airway becomes clearer is tremendous. There's research that shows patients with a lifetime of sleep apnea don't perform at work or school and develop health problems of overweight and heart issues. To see a patient return to me with a crystal-clear airway, enormous amount of energy, able to stay awake in class or at work and have more energy to do sports or other activities in the afternoon and evening is very rewarding.

It's almost like they're a new human being. Their eyebrows and facial expression change to a person excited about life. Their skin color and tone brighten. They seem like they're on fire to enjoy life and usually tell me they had no idea they were miserable and thank me for my diagnosis.

Does a child stop the thumb suck habit because the airway is now fixed? No. They've already developed this habit and there's other things that contributed to it. Airway problems are just one part of the habit. I've not yet in 27 years seen a child stop thumb suck on their own because the airway was just cleared of obstructions.

I've noticed the above in more than 25 years of practice. This has also been noticed by Dr. Leon Treger, a Holistic Dentist, in an article written by Andrea Donsky titled, "Experts say this is why your child sucks their finger or thumb." Dr. Treger stated, studies show that thumb sucking is a child's way to attempt to breathe easier. Thus, thumb sucking "is the body's innate way to establish an airway."

If you suffer with allergies, you know it involves inflammation of the airways and sinuses. Allergies are also intimately associated with inflamed adenoids and enlarged tonsils, two conditions often seen in children, which compromises their ability to breathe well.

Dr. Treger further elaborated, children checked for sensitivities and/or allergies, must get their adenoids and tonsils examined as well. If the sensitivities/allergies are dealt with, children will be able to breathe better and their tonsils and adenoids can reduce in size. Some children may need to have their adenoids and/or tonsils removed.

Other negative problems in the way at school or in the family that will prevent success of the techniques in this book

It's only common sense that if there's a parent alcoholic at home, a drug user, there's domestic violence or arguments exist all the time that the child's not able to focus, is always in fear, nervous and won't be able to concentrate and succeed in the techniques of the thumb sucker buster techniques in this book. Those problems need to be resolved first.

Problems at school from the child harassed by a bully or taunted by others for different things that may or may not be related to the thumb suck. In other words, the thumb sucking was seen by others at school or friends have told others that the thumb suck problem existed that causes unusual relationships at school and taunting.

Or, it was from the child failed at school due to non-usage of dictionaries and went to the next grade level when they really didn't finish the previous grade level that caused the failure. This complex problem needs resolved first.

Yes, with a divorce rate over 50% in the world, it's also hard on children today to focus and do well in school. If the child is exposed to the negative parts of a separation or the beginnings of a divorce will deter the child from success with these easy thumb suck buster techniques that usually work under normal conditions.

Other children in the family or the child's friends thumb suck

In the early stages of the development of these thumb suck buster techniques, I've treated children for the thumb suck habit and found that within one week, the child didn't make much improvement. That's because they copycatted an older brother, sister or a friend in the neighborhood or at school because they somehow had made survival decisions or tried to learn how to live life or respond to life through these people instead of a normal solution to their problem or problems that usually worked instead.

The child assumes it's okay to suck because everyone else does it. This is one of the troubleshooting things I added to the troubleshoot chapter because a lot of these things need to be addressed in the preparation stage before application of the thumb sucker buster techniques.

I even found one child who had given their thumb a name like it was a pet dog and after one week the child didn't perform well and once we discovered this I educated the child that it wasn't a pet and more importantly addressed the fact why the child didn't give a name to all the other fingers and thumbs on both hands and all the toes until the child snapped out of it and realized they didn't have to suck anymore. The child will stop the thumb suck habit within three days with use of these thumb suck buster techniques.

So, yes, you do have to ask the child, do they know someone else that thumb sucks at home, in the neighborhood or they had seen this on TV or they know someone at school.

Take photos of your child when & where they suck their thumb

You'll need these photos later as part of the techniques later in this book. You must get every time and location, day and night the habit's done. If the thumb, finger, toe, pacifier or blanket sucker asks why all the photos, just simply tell them you need a photo.

CHAPTER 6

The Four Types of Thumbsuckers

The four types of thumb suckers are:

1. All the time, day and night.
2. Daytime only.
3. Before bed only.
4. Nighttime only.

Type I: All the time, day and night

These thumb suckers are the hardest to stop. They're a very intense sucker. The reason they're the hardest to stop isn't that they won't stop or my viewpoint that they are hard to stop, it's that it takes so much work to uncover where they do it, when they do it in comparison to the other three. They'll first stop daytime and still do nighttime. Rarely, do I see nighttime stop first to leave daytime to then handle.

When I first meet the child with the parent, I hear they suck all day & night and the mother will usually say this in a very dramatic fashion. I always think to myself that we all have lots of work to do, but I don't show this thought to the parent or mother so that I stay positive for the parent and child. I think this positively since I know they'll stop, that the techniques work in this book and the amount of work by me, the child and the parent doesn't need expressed. That includes no deep sigh or comments as "this is a pretty intense habit you have and will take a lot of work," or "wow, this will take a lot of time."

I very rarely want the input of the mother of where all the locations and when the child sucks because I want the communication to go back and forth between me and the child. So, I tell the mother that I'll ask these questions of the child and she can help me get the child to answer, but not to fill in the blanks.

Often, when the child doesn't respond or fast enough I'll use the question-and-answer technique with the child to illicit a response. For instance, I'll ask, "Do you suck your thumb in the backseat of the car?" The child will say, "Yes." Then ask, "Do you suck your thumb before you go to bed while you lay your head on the pillow?" The child will say, "Yes." Then say, "Do you do it when you come home from school and get on the sofa?" The child will say, "Yes." This question and answer technique makes it smooth and fast.

This starts to open a communication dialogue and establishes a relationship of trust between me and the child. For the first time, they realize that someone understands their problem and won't try to use force, threats or techniques that don't work. They recognize a real true duplication, communication and understanding of their problem and what they must deal with on a day-to-day basis because they really want to stop, but don't understand their problem.

This is one of the most crucial parts of the thumb sucker buster techniques is a child with a problem or habit has someone who really understands what they're day is like and their thought processes are like when they thumb suck. This step can't be left out. I do better to go down a list of questions as stated above rather than have an open-ended question which isn't as effective of, "Can you tell me all the places you suck your thumb?" or "Can you tell me when, day and night, do you suck your thumb?"

There's a difference there and more importantly you won't get all the times and locations because when you question the child with answers, not only does it help them realize you understand their problem, but you'll likely get them to confront these times and places and not forget any of them when they answer you.

Yes, sometimes I have a mother who'll still interject other answers and I complement the mother at that time even though I know she's sits and restrains herself as she listens to the questions and answers go back and forth between myself and the child. Any answer the mom does give, requires me to give a look at the child and ask them, "Does this sound right to you?" so that I don't lose the communication line between myself and the child and to also make sure they confront this extra answer or answers at this preparation stage.

Answers children have given over the past twenty-seven years as places where they suck:

1. Sofa.
2. Car.
3. Closet.
4. Under the bed.
5. On the bed.
6. Backseat of the car.
7. Walk with a parent.
8. Wait for a meal.
9. Watch TV.
10. In the stands at a baseball game.

11. At the mall.
12. In the restaurant booth after a meal.
13. Lazy boy chair.
14. Long road trips.

Type II: Daytime only

You would figure that this type is the easiest to stop, but it's the second hardest one to stop below the all day and night Type I. I find that if a child is awake and thumb sucks at daytime, they're aware that they do it and they decided each time when they do it and those decisions are harder to deal with than the other two types of before bed and nighttime only.

You still want to use the same question and answer technique listed in the Type I thumb sucker. You need to discover when and where in the day the child does this. Keep in mind that if the child goes to school Monday through Friday have different answers than when the child isn't at school on the weekend or on summer vacation.

But, do realize that if they're at camp or they stay with a babysitter or some other scenario exists that full answers and complete answers need found out where and when. This includes when the child stays two to three days at the mother's house and the other days at the father's house in cases of divorce.

So, I make a list each day where the child is, then proceed with each day where they suck and when they suck their thumb.

Type III: Before bed only

Before bedtime only and not while asleep is the easiest of the four to stop. I've found that this person will thumb suck only as a part of a routine to fall asleep. Many of us do different things to get us ready to fall asleep.

Some people eat a Klondike ice cream square bar an hour before sleep like my father did to get their sugar up and then as the sugar level in their blood crashes it makes them tired and then they go to bed. Some people brush their teeth and fold the covers down to have everything ready to fall asleep. Others will read. People exist who I know drink coffee of all things. Some like to take a hot bath. But, it's not just a period before bed that people wind down, but they go through a certain routine like a robot because this routine works for them to fall asleep.

Type IV: Nighttime only and/or before bed

When I interview the child, I ask questions about where and when the thumb suck occurs, I find I must go back and forth with questions of before bed, while sleep and when the child wakes up so I get the full picture of what happens at this time of day for the thumb sucker.

While the parent sits near, I ask the child, "Do you suck your thumb at night?" Most of the time the child states they don't know. Over 50% of the parents state they don't know either. In these situations, I must ask questions as, "Do you go to sleep with your thumb in your mouth?" And, "Do you wake up with it in your mouth?"

There's a section in this book about Band-Aids and sometimes we'll find the child who doesn't know if they suck their thumb at night and the parent doesn't know either that we decide to use Band-Aids applied the same way as in that section of this book and tell the child that to please check the Band-Aids in the morning to see if they're wet that indicates they do suck while asleep. Otherwise, when the child sucks while asleep, sometimes the Band-Aids will wake them up a little bit in the night enough for them to tell me or the parent the next they do suck.

CHAPTER 7

The Power to Decide Process: How to Get a Thumb Sucker to Realize They Already Have the Power to Decide to Stop

The power to decide processes helps the child realize that he can stop his thumb suck habit. The key word here is **DECIDE.** To focus on this word while you do this entire book is where 100% of the success lies. It isn't hope someone will do one or two or three of the processes or other helpful ideas.

The power to decide processes are seven basic EZ techniques:

1. Get the child to see themselves suck in photos taken earlier in this book.
2. Go to the mall with all your friends.
3. Have someone stay over and spend the night that is a celebrity.

4. In front of your class or at a meeting in front of your coworkers.
5. At a birthday party with all your friends.
6. Play baseball, softball or sandlot football with all your friends.
7. Nothing you can do about the past, except to look at it in your mind as if it was photos in a photo album. Now and into the future is how problems are resolved.

The above EZ techniques are simply a technique that falls under one exact precise word, **DICHOTOMY.** Found in the *Business Dictionary,* the definition of dichotomy:

> Division of one thing into two parts, normally differ or oppose each other; the state of being two-fold, have two different components. People discuss the dichotomy of body and soul, men and women, or eastern and western culture. Read more:
> http://www.businessdictionary.com/definition/di chotomy.html

Dichotomy is to look at something and then look at the opposite of that same thing. You'll figure out what you've done and what you'll do whether it's personal, business or in a relationship. Another way to say this is look at how things are and then look at how they're not.

You must compare things in life and when you do the comparison, pick opposites so that your mind can decide quickly. There's no maybe or should be or ought to be or using words while you think that end in "-ing" because if you talk like that then you'll think like that and then you'll never decide. Words that end in "-ing" will make your mind run and run and think and think and nothing will ever get done or decided. Get to the point!

So, yes, the way you talk to the thumb sucker and the way you get the thumb sucker to think differently in their speech and their thought process is to get rid of any words that are maybe and words that end in "-ing". If you don't believe me on this you read a page of information that you wrote five minutes ago with these types of words that are conditional words (should be, may be, ought to be, probably, I'll think about it, running, cooking, working).

Then, ask yourself, "What I just read, is so indecisive, a bore, a waste of my time, got nothing done and nothing decided." Then, you'll realize the power of words not only in what you write, in what you say to others, but these words are in your thoughts and this alone will change you and the thumb sucker in front of you for life.

With the power to decide processes, you get the thumb sucker to also see that they don't thumb suck at certain times and locations and that when they don't suck they need to carry that same attitude, emotion and action to when they do suck at other times and locations.

Don't forget to tell the thumb sucker that they know it's not okay to suck at those times and locations, but without use of sinful or bad words, get the point across in gentle expressions that they know it's also not okay to thumb suck just because no one's around and get them to make an agreement with you about these times and locations.

Power to Decide Processes:

1. **Get the child to see themselves suck in photos taken earlier in this book:**

Show the sucker each picture in the front of this book of the different types of thumb suckers. After each picture is shown, ask the sucker what does this person look like. The sucker needs to answer, baby.

Then, show each picture of the sucker you took earlier in preparation to work with the sucker to stop and get the sucker to see for themselves this matches their previous answer above that it looks like a baby. Don't give them the answer; help them or give hints to get them to originate it on their own.

Please don't print these photos out and put them around the house or on the refrigerator. You don't need negative reminders to get the sucker to stop.

2. **Go to the mall with all your friends:**

Get the thumb sucker to imagine a trip to the mall this weekend on Saturday to see all their friends. Ask, "Will you suck your thumb in front of your friends at the food court?" Of course, they'll say, "No."

Then, tell them, "You'll walk around the mall with your parents where other people will see you suck." "Will you suck your thumb as you shop?" They'll say, "No."

Then, ask him, "Why won't you do it?" They'll say, "It'll embarrass me and I don't want people to think I'm a baby." And, you acknowledge him and let him know, "Good, you made the right decision." Notice that you acknowledged his power of decision. Let them know that they're in control of this and that you, not like their parents, won't control the situation or demand them to decide, but rather they'll decide.

So, with all this in mind, tell them, "Now that you decided to stop your habit, you must realize that you do have the power in your mind to stop thumb suck. If you can hang at the mall all day and night for twenty-four hours and all your friends are there, you won't suck your thumb for twenty-four hours, will you?" They'll say, "No, I won't."

This uplifts me so much compared to many other techniques in the history of thumb sucking. Psychologists never figured it out and basically got it wrong. Most of their techniques use transference which basically has a person control a habit or overcome a problem by living their life through the therapists. The patient never can resolve things totally on their own without dependency on the therapist and is hooked to the therapist for life and can't make any decisions on their own.

So, if you wonder if this is psychology or some form of hypnotism – NO! I don't play that game or any of those techniques because they have totally failed in the past. Plus, the labels that psychologists have given thumb suckers in the past don't match what I found and is another reason why they failed ... label a child with a diagnosis of big medical words or terms.

3. Have someone stay over and spend the night that's a celebrity.

Ask the thumb sucker for a list of three famous people they'd like to meet. If they can't think of someone, help them with categories as singers, movie stars and sports players. You'll get awesome answers from the thumb sucker. If it's a child, look over at the parent and notice they didn't know this about their child answer's.

I've had answers as Michael Jordan, the singer Usher, Justin Bieber, politicians, Dale Earnhardt, Jr., Madonna and Britney Spears. Then, ask them to pick one of the three.

Tell them to imagine that tonight this person will arrive at 6:00 PM to have dinner with you and the family at the dining room table and they'll spend the night at your home.

Then, ask them, "Will you suck your thumb at the dinner table in front of them?" They'll state, "No." Then, ask, "Will you suck your thumb before you go to bed or while you sleep because they'll sleep on your bed while you sleep on the sofa and they may get up in the middle of the night and see you?' They'll state, "No."

Ask them, "Why won't you suck?" They'll state, "They don't want the celebrity to see them suck and think less of them." Ask, "That's awesome. So, if this celebrity is with you 24 hours a day you won't suck your thumb, right?" They'll say, "No."

State, "You then have the power to decide to carry the same thought that you have right now in your mind and carry that over to every minute of the day and night and put that in right now to decide not to ever suck your thumb again."

While you move your head vertically up and down, indicates a yes, but don't say anything, wait for the child to say, "Yes." You'll literally wake them up and shift them over from to suck to the other side of the dichotomy to not suck decision.

4. In front of your class or at a meeting in front of your coworkers.

Tell them, imagine you're in front of your class at school and you tell them about the weekend you had. While you tell them the weekend story you try to decide whether to put your thumb in your mouth for them to see. You don't because they'll laugh at you and think you're dog meat.

I found out that the words dog meat is cool to use with a child since that is the sort of language they use. It'll cause them to laugh because they know what those words mean and they think it's cool that you used those words or description with them and not seem like some "old" adult who gives advice they don't want to hear or tries to control them or have a must do tone to what they say.

Ask them, "Why won't you suck?" They'll state they don't want the classmates or coworkers to see them thumb suck and they'd think less of them. Ask, "That's awesome. So, if these classmates or coworkers were with you 24 hours a day you won't suck your thumb, right?" They'll state, "No."

State, "You then have the power to decide to carry the same thought that you have right now in your mind and carry that over to every minute of the day and night and put that in right now to decide not to ever suck your thumb again."

While you move your head vertically up and down to encourage a yes answer, but don't say anything, wait for the child to say, "Yes."

5. At a birthday party with all your friends.

Tell them, you're now at a surprise birthday party. 20 friends are there and they all brought presents. Ask, "Will you suck your thumb?" They'll answer, "No."

So, imagine the birthday party goes on for seven days in a row and you don't need to sleep. Will you be able to not suck your thumb for seven days, 24 hours a day? They'll state, "Yes."

So, you do have the power to decide when to do it and when not to do it, "Yes?" They'll say, "Yes."

6. **While play your favorite sport … baseball, soccer.**

Ask, "What is your favorite sport?" Get very exact details on this subject and really let him know that you care about their day-to-day life routines. What I mean by this is, for example if a boy, you may find out that he skateboards, but he loves to play baseball more. He tells you he plays the position of a first baseman and he loves to hit the ball. So, you ask him, "While you play first base do you suck your thumb?" He'll say, "No."

"How about when you sit on the bench while you wait your turn to bat?" He'll say, "No."

"Do you think you'll play baseball 24 hours a day if you don't have to sleep?" So, "You do have the ability to decide not to suck your thumb if you think you'll play baseball 24 hours a day?" He'll state, "Yes."

7. **Nothing you can do about the past, except to look at it in your mind as if it was photos in a photo album. Now and into the future is how problems are resolved.**

Ask, "Can you do anything about last week or last year or two years ago?" They'll state, "No."

"Can you do anything about something in five minutes from now?" They'll state, "Yes."

"Can you do anything about something next week or next year?" They'll state, "Yes."

Ask, "What's the point to all of this?" They'll state, "There's nothing you can do about the past … only the present and future." Tell them, "Very good."

Ask, "Can you do anything about sucking your thumb this morning, or last night or yesterday or last week or last year?" They'll state, "No."

Ask, "Why's that?" They'll state, "It's only in my memory or my mind. But, I'm here right now and I have the future."

This perfectly sets up the next scenario.

Ask, "You have the right to make things go right and do things correctly and start right now, right?" They'll state, "Yes."

"You also have the right to forgive yourself because you made a mistake and others will forgive you since everyone has made mistakes. Correct?" They'll state, "Yes."

The key statement right now is to tell them, "You have my permission to start fresh right now and never thumb suck again and pretend that it never happened since it's now only a memory. Is that okay with you?" They'll state, "Yes."

I tell them, "Awesome!"

Last Step of Power to Decide Processes:

(Note to the reader: This is the hardest part of these processes is to get to this point.)

So, you ask the thumb sucker, "Again, do you realize that you have the power to stop anything, start anything, control this habit and can just let it go and never do it again?" They'll say, "Yes, I have the ability to stop suck my thumb."

Then, ask them, "Do you want to stop suck your thumb?" They'll say, "Yes, I do want to stop."

Tell them, "Great! Let's move on to the next step to help you in different places and times so you can help yourself not get in the situation where you feel like you had to suck. We'll now handle the urges that pop up day to day and how to make those urges go away. Sound good?" They'll say, "Yes."

CHAPTER 8

Break Routines, Times & Locations, Where the Child Sucked in the Past

This chapter is broken into two parts:

1. Repeat a short version of where the thumb sucker sucks and where they don't to set them up for part two.
2. Break up the routine, time and locations where the child sucks in part one.

Part 1: Repeat a short version of where the thumb sucker sucks and where they don't to set them up for part two.

Now, you'll get the child to go into a different process with use of dichotomies of routines, times and locations. Ask the child, "Tell me where you suck your thumb." If they don't say anything go ahead and help coach him along. Ask, "Do you do it at home on the sofa when you come home from school when you're a little tired? They'll say, "Yes or no."

Ask, "Do you do it in the closet where no one can see you?" They'll say, "Yes or no."

"Have you done it at home on a Sunday afternoon when you're tired and bored with nothing to do?" They'll say, "Yes or no."

"Do you suck your thumb in the back seat of a car on a vacation trip or for a short trip to the grocery store or to get ice cream?" They'll say, "Yes or no."

"Do you suck your thumb at night when you go to bed?" They'll say, "Yes or no." If they say, "Yes," ask, "Do you suck before you fall asleep to help you go to sleep?" They'll answer, "Yes or no."

These questions are very important because there are different ways to handle each different type of thumb sucker. Some suck only at night, some suck only in the day and there are ones that suck day and night. Each type of sucker is treated differently.

Tell them, "Now let's go into all the places where you don't suck your thumb."

"Do you do it in front of your class when you're at school?" They'll say, "No."

"Do you suck your thumb when you go out to dinner with your parents?" They'll say, "No."

"How about in front of your friends at a birthday party, do you suck your thumb?" They'll say, "No."

So, go through all these times where they suck and not suck. Go back through them again where you find where they do and where they don't. Then, you'll get the most marvelous response from the child when you ask, "Do you really need to suck your thumb?" They'll say, "No."

Part 2: Break Routines and Locations Associated with Where the Child Sucked in the Past

Sofa:

To do this, you'll basically make alterations in locations the habit is done. For instance, the easiest solution for the child who comes home and gets on the sofa in front of the TV and sucks is to have him sit and not lay on the sofa. Better yet, we prefer them to be in a different chair and not lay down.

Remind them that to lie down and/or to take a nap at their age isn't good that we don't want them to take a nap. If they're tired is one thing, but if they don't need a nap, then don't take one. It's best for them to go outside and extrovert and take a walk or shoot basketball hoops.

Before Sleep:

Suck before bedtime in the bed is a routine. Tell the thumb sucker they made the decision to stop suck today and their mom will allow them to stay up an hour later tonight. For the next week, you want the thumb sucker very tired so that when they go to sleep they'll crash and burn and not even think about the thumb suck as part of the equation to fall asleep.

Something that helps the "go to bed sucker" is to have someone come in the room with a chair beside the bed and give the thumb sucker a back massage. Don't get on the bed since when the thumb sucker falls asleep and you get off the bed you'll wake the them up.

Have the thumb sucker face away from you on the bed and gently rub their back and legs and in about ten to fifteen minutes they'll get sleepy and then the massager can make the massage more into a gentle rub. After the massager can tell the thumb sucker has gone to sleep, they can leave the room and not wake the thumb sucker since the massager isn't on the bed. The massager must do this for a week if the thumb sucker's a heavy thumb sucker before sleep.

Back seat of the car:

The same thing goes for the backseat of a car. We prefer the child in the front seat for thirty days. If he must be in the backseat they can't lie down and keep them pre-occupied with a video on the phone or a video player.

3:00 PM to 6:00 PM phenomenon:

I tell every thumb sucker that we eat between 7:00 AM and 8:00 AM and then four hours later, we eat at 12 o'clock noon. That's only four to five hours. Then, we don't eat dinner until 6-8 o'clock at night. That's a six to eight hours gap of time. The problem is that around 3-4 o'clock PM people get hungry and get tired.

I noticed that in South America they have Siesta where in many small towns a church bell rings and everyone stops and lays down. In England, they have tea and crumpets at 4:00 PM. This breaks up the routine, gives a rest and nutrition or snack to hold them over 'til dinner.

The thumb sucker must do this to counter the 3-6 o'clock PM phenomenon. I recommend a protein snack eaten once they walk in the door from school and not allowed to go lay down on the sofa, but to go back outside and shoot basketball hoops, walk, play to get fresh air or exercise. This will take their mind off their habit and break up the routine to watch TV, get on the sofa and then the thumb makes its way into the mouth.

Between 3:00 pm and dinner this must occur. Unless they work on their goal and creativity from another chapter. No video games or TV allowed at this period.

Snacks mustn't include cakes, cookies, ice cream or other sugar products that will make them sluggish and more tired. Plus, those foods tend to ruin the appetite for dinner. If the thumb sucker is overweight they must focus on exercise in the gym or other means. An apple or pear that has fiber and gives bulk to the stomach to not feel hungry is best.

Finally:

So, what happens here is to break up the thumb sucker's routine. We don't want the thumb sucker to get into situations just like a person who wants to quit cigarette smoking. The person who no longer smokes won't do well if cigarettes were all around him at a sports bar to watch his favorite sports team as their friends puff away. The same thing goes with the thumb sucker is that we don't want them in any situation or location that will trigger the habit to begin again.

CHAPTER 9

Confront Your Age Technique

The first thing you must do is get the child who's five years old or older to realize that they're not two or under anymore. To do this, go through a series of questions.

Ask them, "Do you know what age a baby or infant is?" They'll guess. You reply with, "It's up to age 1."

Ask them, "Do you know that you're not supposed to suck past the age of two?" They'll say, "No."

"Do you know that sucking is for babies up to age one?" They'll say, "No."

Have the child now raise their right hand and show you how old they are with their fingers. If the child is five years old, they'll have five fingers shown on one hand. Now, ask the child, "Up to what age are you able to suck your thumb as a baby? Show me on your left hand how many fingers is your answer." The child will put up one finger on the left-hand. Be sure that both hands have both answers shown so the child will confront the age difference.

Now you'll switch to analogies. First ask them, "Will it be okay if your mother came to school with you in the first grade and sit there all day long in those small chairs you sit in and take the same courses you take?" They'll say, "No."

Next, ask them, "Will it be okay for your dad to be dressed up in the same outfit to play soccer as you do and come be on the field with you just like the other kids?" They'll say, "No."

"So, imagine your parents come to school or play with you on the soccer field and that it will look too weird to do this because they're too old to do those things. Will it be okay for you to suck your thumb if you're not supposed to do it past the age of one?" They'll say, "No, I was supposed to stop."

Say to the child, "So, when someone sees you suck your thumb at age five or whatever age you are, what do you think they think?" Most of the time the child will state, "They think I'm a baby or it's a little weird that this older child sucks their thumb." I'm amazed how many children right there will give that answer.

And, last, it's always best to end with a very important question after the correct answers have been given above, "Do you feel it's okay to suck your thumb at your age anymore?" 100% of the time the child will state, "No." Then, you can ask them, "Will you like to be able to stop and never do it again?" The child will always say, "Yes."

CHAPTER 10

Funny Story about the First Patient Who Stopped the Thumb Suck Habit

Let me tell the story about the first thumb sucker who came to my office that helped me develop what's in this book. She was six years old and the daughter of a dental hygienist.

The dental hygienist stated that she was embarrassed by the fact that she didn't get her child to stop thumb suck because she worked in the dental field and had some sort of diplomatic immunity because of her status. She felt she was inherently able to have figured out how to have stopped it.

Interestingly, many parents feel guilty as this dental hygienist that they can't stop their children from habits as this one. She had tried numerous things to get her to stop. I worked with the child numerous visits until the child stopped. Back then it took numerous visits to address different topics that were beta tested where today everything can be done in a one-hour visit.

In one month, the child had officially stopped. The mother came forward and stated that I did an awesome job, but she was further embarrassed to tell me that her child also sucked her large right toe.

My first response of course was, "Why didn't you tell me?" She stated, "I'm embarrassed and I thought that she'd stop the toe habit when she stopped the thumb habit." I then asked, "Is there anything else that I should know about?" She said, "No." And, we all laughed.

We did the same techniques all over again and she stopped her toe suck. Then, I found out when I talked to the child ... and the mother didn't think anything about it ... that she also sucked a blanket. She took the corner of a small blanket and folded it up into a knot and sucked on it.

We then had to go through the technique a third time to get her off that and it was at that time we noticed the changes in her as mentioned in this book about how a child doesn't seem like a baby any more and more importantly they don't even talk like one. Yes, many thumb suckers not only suck as a one-year-old, but act and talk like one ... yet this magically disappears when the thumb habit vanishes.

This was such a reward for me to see the mother state that she noticed all these changes as if her daughter had caught up to her real age in a matter of one to two months and, yet the child welcomed this and didn't resist nor had problems with it.

CHAPTER 11

Changes Noticed in Patients, Adults & Children after Stop the Thumb Suck Habit

Changes I've noticed in thumb suckers are numerous. The biggest one is their communication changes from a sort of baby talk to normal talk. You won't spot the change right away, but there will be a noticeable difference in four weeks.

Parents of children who thumb suck tell me of the change as quick as one week. Adult thumb suckers will tell me their co-workers and friends tell them of the change.

I noticed a more dramatic change in the thumb sucker myself as I only see them once a week versus the people in the thumb sucker's life sees them sometimes all day, seven days a week and not notice the change day to day. But, when a parent tells me they do notice the change in their child it makes the work done with their child well worth it. Also, the rewarding feeling I get is to see that I helped their child change and for them to have a better quality of life.

The communication changes from a sort of baby talk to more complete sentences. The communication steers more towards a desire to have a conversation and not to just answer questions. They'll start to originate new topics for discussion.

You'll also notice another change in the thumb sucker's behavior. A child thumb sucker even as old as nine or 10 won't do things to get attention, cry to get things they want or other things like a baby does and will start to act more like an adult. I've seen changes in a seven-year-old who acted like a two-year-old. They always cried and threw temper tantrums. Within one week they acted as a seven-year-old.

Child thumb suckers will stop collection of stuff animals if they're 10 or older. They'll communicate more with their siblings. It's like a flower bulb that now opens and blossoms right in front of your eyes.

In teenage and adult thumb suckers, I noticed a change in hairstyle and makeup. The amazement and surprise I get on a weekly basis from my thumb suck patients catches me off-guard all the time. Often, the change will cause me to think back to when I first met the patient and I didn't know an outpoint of their characteristic, mannerism or speech was out; but now I do spot it.

While you help a thumb sucker, don't be surprised to get the same thought I get every time I help one, that I say to myself, it's like the thumb sucker was stuck at the age they first started to thumb suck. And, these techniques unstick them, and they come up to present time. Don't tell the thumb sucker this thought, but do tell them you understand if they happen to originate that they feel this way. Of course, there are a few who never say their speech changed even though I noticed it.

I just let it be and notice my own personal satisfaction that I helped an adult or child thumb sucker make this change. To help someone make a difference in their life is the highest reward in life. There's an old cliché that to help someone will cause a flow of help back to you many times in mysterious and unknown ways when you flow help outwards to others.

Don't push the change. Not all children and adults change at the same speed. You must give them a chance to grow out of this problem because the change may be too drastic for them to handle. And, you need to complement the thumb sucker as further changes occur and let them know you notice the communication changes. Tell them you're so proud of them for the decision to stop the thumb suck habit and the changes that have occurred with their communication.

Try to avoid a complement worded "that they finally grew up" because that may come across wrong to the thumb sucker as if they acted as a baby in the past. Don't say, "I notice that now that you no longer thumb suck that you don't talk like a baby anymore." That will only make the thumb sucker wonder how bad they were when they thumb sucked. Also, don't try to force the child or adult to change if they still do baby-like communication or mannerisms like a two-year-old.

We can only encourage them and gently talk with them, but don't force this especially in the first thirty days of these techniques. Once the child has reached their thirty straight days of no suck, I haven't seen a child go back to the habit.

If a traumatic thing occurs in their life that reverts the thumb sucker back to the habit, then they must go through the techniques again. No comments by anyone to the thumb sucker of frustration or sympathy are given; just do the techniques again.

CHAPTER 12

New Goals & Creativity

Psychologists got it all wrong in the past that a thumb sucker is introverted. I've found that they're extroverted, bored and don't create enough. I recommend projects towards goals, do something creative and learn something new.

Learn something new as:

- Play a musical instrument as a piano or a six-string guitar. Be sure to keep in mind that if a child or someone has never played a musical instrument they must learn how to play something simple first as a six-string guitar or a simple plastic flute until they read sheet music and get lessons, or they buy a DVD online that teaches them quickly.
- Golf lessons.
- Learn a foreign language with Rosetta Stone or other means.
- Art lessons.
- Sail lessons.
- Sing lessons.
- Write music and songs.
- Write books.
- Write poetry.
- Other creative things.

If the child thumb sucks between the age of five and seven, it is crucial to have them shift thought processes to a sport or to learn a musical instrument. It may even lead them to something that's not only fun, but a career.

Tiger Woods started golf at age two. Most thumb suckers are bored and don't create enough. Two things I just stated:

- One is bored ... means nothing to do.
- But, I find the second of not create enough is the most important.

When you decide to do something for the child to extrovert them, you don't want them just to go and shoot basketball hoops. I prefer them to create something that they can see as a real product from their mind and for others to see.

Example of this is draw with a charcoal pencil. At age 6, I used charcoal pencils to draw historical houses as Mount Vernon, home of George Washington. The child can either copy what he sees in front of him or from a picture on the internet or draw something from the mind that may or may not be a real object.

When and how do you start goals and creativity for the thumb sucker? Now. After you present the techniques in this book, the last step is to start goals and creativity.

Ask the thumb sucker five goals they want to achieve in the next six months, next year and in 10 years. Write their answers down. They'll need help later to map out the steps of each goal and write down target dates to get the steps done. Life is about the past, now and the future. We learn from the past and we can see it in our mind and it affects us now and in the future, but if we focus on now and the future and get away from the past thoughts, we'll achieve things faster. At this point you must get the thumb sucker to think about creativity rather than to thumb suck.

Ask the thumb sucker five things they'd like to learn that are fun. You can give suggestions in a positive manner. Ask, "Do you want to play a musical instrument like a saxophone or a six-string guitar?" If the thumb sucker can't come up with any answers, then you'll have to pick something that they can do that's easy while they take their mind off their habit and come up with ideas of their own.

If they pick something that requires to read or listen to new words on the Internet, video or DVD, be sure they know how to use a dictionary and how to recognize words and symbols. To use a dictionary, they'll realize they can learn anything.

If money is a concern and it isn't feasible to do lessons, get creative. I've found Esteban's complete Guitar course for beginners online for $12.99. Esteban guitar for $50-99.

This will be one of the rewards you receive from the thumb sucker is to deliver these techniques to the thumb sucker and get them to create. To help them stop the habit is one thing, but to help someone find their creative path in life is another.

CHAPTER 13

Reminder Positive Tools, Not Negative Punishment Tools

The key is positive presentation to the thumb sucker, not the tool itself

Always tell the thumb sucker that, "You need some extra help. Nothing you'll experience is punishment and is only a reminder to help remind you to not suck your thumb. Nothing you'll experience is intended to make you feel bad and if you do block that out of your mind.

Tell them that no one will know that they're in thumb suck treatment. It's none of their business anyway.

Stay positive in your mannerism and the words you use because the positive presentation is 37% of the reason why the below tools work and not the tool itself. Years ago, there was a study with a medical pill versus a sugar pill and two groups of patients stated that they got well from the sugar pill and didn't know the pill wasn't the medical pill. The placebo pill, because it was presented the same way as the medical pill proved that the presentation alone will allow the patient to feel better about their problem.

Use words as, "I've heard they work very well." "No one will know you're in treatment with use of these." "You'll do very well." "These are easy." "They don't even hurt."

Band-Aids

I always find out first if the thumb sucker has tried Band-Aids. If they have, tell them that this will be totally different and it's a small part of the overall techniques.

Night-time Only Sucker

Band-Aids will be wet in the morning if the thumb sucker has them on their thumb before bed and they suck at night. I recommend they be placed two hours before bed so they aren't focused on them when they're about to go to sleep.

Place the Band-Aids with the cotton on the inside part of the thumb away from the nail at the first knuckle. A second Band-Aid is placed over the first one halfway up towards the nail, but be sure neither Band-Aid is too tight or causes too much pressure. Have the child bend their thumb with the Band-Aids on to check if they're too tight. Yet, you don't want them to fall off because their too loose.

And yes, if the thumb sucker sucks a second thumb or finger, these will also need Band-Aids.

Daytime Sucker

The Band-Aids must be on all day long. If they go to school or work, they need to keep a small baggie in their pocket with four extra Band-Aids. Tell them that they don't want to set themselves up for failure just because they get one wet when they go to wash their hands at the bathroom and they don't have a new one to put on.

Tell them that if anyone asked about their Band-Aids, they can make something up as they had a paper cut, it's there to help them remind them of something or whatever excuse and the other person will usually move on to talk about something else.

If it's summertime and they're at the pool or beach, they must take extra Band-Aids to put back on when they get wet. The same applies for sports.

Simple Band-Aids Rules

Tell the thumb sucker the Band-Aids aren't punishment and that they're only a reminder to help them stop sucking. Tell them you won't be happy with them and will become very disappointed if they suck after removal of the Band-Aids. If they want to suck it must be with the Band-Aids on. They must learn that to take them off to suck means that they didn't try one-hundred percent.

Next, tell the thumb sucker, "We have one more rule. If you suck with the Band-aid on or off, you must suck each finger and thumb on both hands one at a time for a minute each. The other fingers and thumb get lonely and it's not fair to give all of your attention to this one thumb."

I notice that to apply this rule does three things for the thumb sucker:

1) First, it gets them out of their routine to suck the same thumb over and over and will help break the robotic habit, circuit or automatic routine they've established.
2) Second, it does a mind reversal trick, since now you've told them it's okay to suck when their parents, friends, and yes, even themselves have stated to stop. The

same sort of thing happened when my own father caught me in high school with a liquor bottle for a party.

A friend dropped it off in the mailbox. My mother decided to put mail in the mailbox the night before instead of the next morning. She took the pint to my father. I expected to be scolded, but my dad did this reversal technique on me. He told me he was disappointed that I didn't come to him to get drinks and that he would in the future. This took all the fun out of the game to get liquor in the future; I no longer desired alcohol at events.

3) Third, to suck each finger a minute each is nine minutes that they won't suck the "thumb culprit" and will shift attention away to something else.

Agreement:

"I agree that I'll:

1. **Not remove the Band-Aids.**
2. **Suck my thumb with the Band-Aid on if I must suck.**
3. **Suck all other eight fingers and the other thumb one minute each if I suck my thumb."**

I get the thumb sucker to give me a handshake after I say the above agreement. If they hesitate to make the agreement or handshake, repeat the agreement until they give a firm acknowledgement and handshake with you.

Final notes about Band-Aids

You'll want to take the thumb sucker to the store and let them select the Band-Aids they want to wear. Children under five like this and usually will select ones with cartoons. Be sure to try the Band-Aid before you leave the store since many clear ones don't have strong glue and will come off easily.

Don't mix other techniques with the ones in this book. For instance, don't apply hot sauces or nail polish because those techniques don't work, and they only make the thumb sucker feel bad. Some parents have tried rubbing alcohol and other chemicals to make the thumb not taste good, but these also don't work, or the child will simply wash them off the thumb.

Another Reminder Positive Tool

I've had success with use of a patient Hawley orthodontic retainer that's used after braces are removed to hold the teeth in place. This is the old-fashioned design with plastic in the roof of the mouth and I place four tiny U-shaped studs in the plastic that aren't visible to the public. When the thumb sucker places the thumb in the mouth they hit the studs that reminds them to get the thumb out of their mouth and to not suck.

What's nice about this is that it's removable. I never treated a thumb suck patient with a glue-in device, crib or rake with sharp spurs. These don't handle the problem of the patient to make the decision to stop and it comes across as punishment. Removable devices are more accepted since they're removed to brush, floss and eat meals. It comes in different colors.

Thumb Guard, Mittens or Gloves

There's a company that makes a plastic cover with Velcro that fits over the thumb. The same can be done with a mitten or glove. I have great success with Band-Aids and the techniques in this book and don't resort to these bigger devices. I'm not against them; I just get the result without them.

CHAPTER 14

Negative Punishment Reminder Tools Not to Use Sauces

Sauces don't work because they don't last long, constantly must be applied and makes the thumb sucker feel bad about themselves. I never had to use or recommend them.

Sauces include:

- Lemon
- Vinegar
- Tabasco sauce
- Cayenne pepper
- Hot pepper
- Soap
- Curry
- Salt
- Others

Verbal threats or physical cues

These don't work and only worsens the relationship between the person who gives them and the thumb sucker.

Then, when they try the techniques in this book, the relationship will be damaged enough that the techniques don't work.

Even physical cues of the way a parent looked unhappily at a child in the past in an effort to stop the habit, although nothing was said, was a form of communication the child stored in the memory as negative connotations.

This form of negative reminder doesn't work.

Nail polish

I've found these don't work because they don't remind enough. Most the time the thumb sucker will put the thumb in the mouth and not look at it. Or, it's night-time and the color of the nail polish isn't visible to remind the child not to suck. There are some nail polishes that don't taste good, but we're back to the theory of sauces again as stated above which I don't recommend and haven't had success with.

Jokes to use a knife or cigar cutter

To tell a child you'll cut their thumb off is drastic. The child will believe the parent and the fear instilled will be hard to remove. The biggest point here is that you won't allow the child to make the decision to stop which is the most powerful part of these techniques. And, it's a punishment drive technique to threaten a child to cut off their thumb so that they won't be able to suck anymore.

There's Heinrich Hoffman's 1845 bedtime classic Struwwelpeter of snip off thumb in Germany.

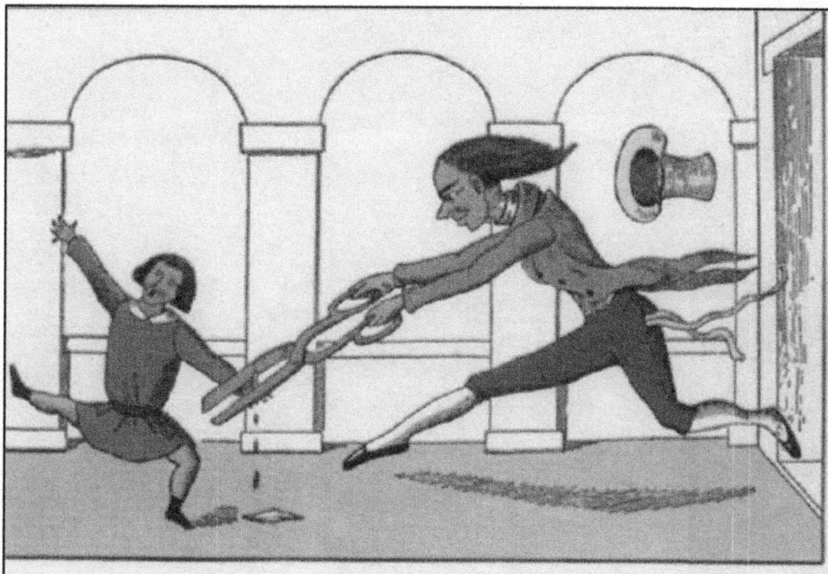

The door flew open, in he ran,
The great, long, red-legg'd scissor-man.
Oh! children, see! the tailor's come
And caught out little Suck-a-Thumb.
Snip! Snap! Snip! the scissors go;
And Conrad cries out — Oh! Oh! Oh!
Snip! Snap! Snip! They go so fast,
That both his thumbs are off at last.

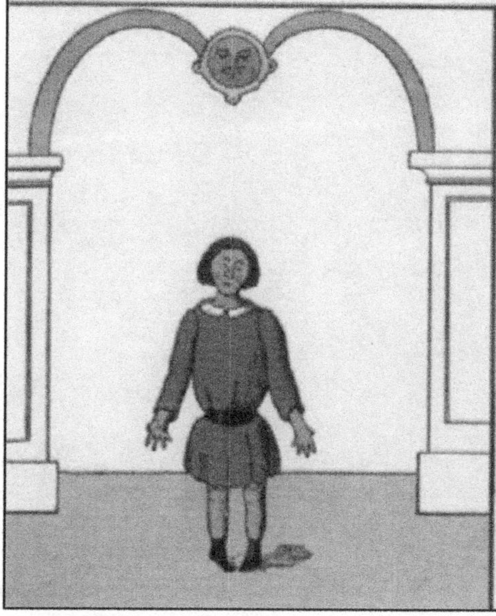

Mamma comes home; there Conrad stands,
And looks quite sad, and shows his hands, —
"Ah!" said Mamma "I knew he'd come
To naughty little Suck-a-Thumb."

CHAPTER 15

Reward System to Help the Thumb Sucker Get to Their Goal: To Stop the Thumb Suck Habit & Final Quick Steps before You End Session with the Thumb Sucker

Reward system

All goals in life need a reward system. To stop the thumb suck habit is the goal. Treatment time is four weeks. Each week a reward needs to be decided by the thumb sucker. A one week, two week, three week and four week reward with the fourth week designated as the final reward is written on the same day the techniques are administered.

A reward system always works with me and my patients. I remember myself as a third grader every time I got a hundred on my spelling test, I earned a gold star and at the end of the year I had the most gold stars and received a reward. A reward system needs mini rewards with the final reward that equates to breakdown of barriers towards any goal.

The reward system needs to be brought up in front of the child thumb sucker while the parent is there. If an adult thumb sucker, they need to write on paper what they'll reward themselves with.

The person who applies these techniques to a child thumb sucker will state in front of the parent that you want the parent to set up a reward system with the child on the way home to start when you get home tonight. Don't let this wait until tomorrow.

Tell the child or adult thumb sucker that they'll fill out a calendar card with checkmarks each full day they don't suck to have them confront their habit. Place it on the refrigerator door where everyone can see it. Instead of a calendar card, a calendar on the refrigerator that has squares for each day can be used.

Each morning, put a check or an S in the square for the previous day and night. If you touched your thumb to your mouth even for a second that's an S and you must start the 30 days again. They must get thirty days in a row of checkmarks to be finished with this technique. Yes, it'll frustrate you when this happens.

The first week reward needs to be a small item as a pair of tennis shoes. It's crucial to not allow the parent to buy the child other things. Certain times of the year it's hard to do the reward system. For instance, when school starts in the fall a parent must buy clothes. Then, there's Christmas, birthdays, etc. You mustn't buy anything except an ice cream cone every now and then; not large materialistic things.

Whether you're a parent of a child thumb sucker or an adult thumb sucker who chooses the rewards, the size or cost of the reward isn't always related to the success of these techniques. I'll tell you a story where a child came back to visit me in one week and stopped the thumb habit. The child told me the four different rewards with the final reward a pony. I took the parent aside and told them they didn't have to do this, but I learned something. The parent stated they live on a farm and planned the pony weeks before the start of the thumb suck treatment.

So, if you already know some things that your child needs you can turn them into rewards. Especially, if you don't want to have to get those same things and come up with separate rewards; it'll all work out in your favor. That wasn't the end of the story. Six months later, the parent told me that they had to sell the pony because the child didn't know how hard the work was to maintain the pony with daily chores to clean the stall, feed the horse and more. But, we got rid of the thumb.

Then, decide what the reward will be for the second week, the third week and then the fourth. It's best to tell the child what week one, two, three and the final forth week awards right after the thumb suck processes in this book have been done. The final award needs to be the ultimate prize.

If a child or adult sees something over the next thirty days and wants something different for one of the rewards, it's okay to switch, but try not to.

After application of these techniques you must see the thumb sucker once a week, but it's best every three to four days. You must monitor them. They must bring their thumb suck calendar card or calendar from the refrigerator. Always draw a happy face on their card to let them know you're happy with their performance and applaud them for excellent cooperation.

If you don't see them every three to four days or at least once a week they'll relapse and go back to the habit and you'll have to start the whole process all over again. Also, the parent may need some help and encouragement. You may find the child or adult won't keep the Band-Aids on their thumb at school or work.

Final quick step before you end the first session with the thumb, finger, toe, pacifier or blanket sucker

After thorough study of this book and after you practice the techniques before they are applied to the thumb sucker, you'll reach the final step within sixty minutes. If you spend more time than this, you'll lose the attention of the child.

Below are the final five things to do:

1) Do the handshake while you state to the thumb sucker, "You agree hundred percent not to take the Band-Aids off and suck each finger thirty seconds each for every time you suck your thumb."
2) Tell the thumb sucker to call you in 24 hours, not the mother. The mother is in the background while you state this to the child. Tell the thumb sucker, "When you call I want you to tell me that you didn't suck your thumb and you feel it has stopped."
3) Tell them that you want to see them in 4 to 6 days for a quick 15-minute visit to check if any urges, problems or thoughts exist.
4) Remind them they must get thirty straight days of checkmarks on their calendar before they can consider their thumb suck habit totally gone.

5) Tell them, "I'm very proud of you right now that you made the decision to stop your thumb suck habit and I know your mom is also proud of you. Good luck!"

CHAPTER 16

Sample: Begin to End Treatment of a First Session Child Thumb Sucker

Present in the room today is Susie and her mom. Susie is six years old and has begun first grade three months ago. Susie sits in a chair and faces me about three feet apart. The mother has been told to only answer questions that are directed at her and not to help the child. She sits behind and to the left of the child so that the child can turn and see the mother if they want to.

The back of the throat has been checked and there are no large tonsils and there's no breathing problems or dark rings around the child's eyes. The child sleeps well and there aren't home problems.

Also, mom had her eat protein food and not much sugar since it was 4 o'clock in the afternoon and she wasn't tired. You don't want to do this if the child's hungry, sleepy or had a rough day. Reschedule if things aren't perfect.

Dr. Fox: "Susie, I'm here to discuss with you about your thumb suck habit. You do realize you have one, right?"

Susie: "Dr. Fox I already know that it hurt my teeth and I want to stop. I know my mom is frustrated with me that I haven't stopped, and she has tried many things."

Dr. Fox:" I want you to look at the pictures in the front of this book and notice these people suck different things. What does this picture look like?"

Suzie: "A baby."

Dr. Fox: "Great. (Continued to show 4 more photos with the same answers). Now, here are some photos of you do the same. What does this photo look like?"

Susie: "A baby."

Dr. Fox: "Very good. I've shown you these photos of others and you to help you realize that you need to see yourself with this habit because many times I find a person with this habit only sees things through their eyes and not from a distance and many times they don't see themselves do this habit.

I want you to put all the things that seem negative to you, in the past up to this point, not in your thoughts anymore. Your mom loves you and has tried to help and sometimes things like this can get frustrate you and her. It can lessen your relationship between the two of you and affect the way you talk to each other. Don't you agree?"

Susie: "Yes."

Dr. Fox: "I really believe if you want to stop you will and that is why your mom wants me to help you. Will you like to stop?"

Susie: "Yes."

Dr. Fox: "Everything we're about to do over the next half an hour to one hour is positive talk only. If anything I say to you sounds like it's negative or I make you feel bad, I want you to raise your right hand. I'll stop immediately and ask how are you and you must tell me what it is that I said that's negative because nothing from this point onward will be said to you in that tone or manner.

Also, I want you to know that from this point forward your mother won't say anything negative to you. This includes on the way home today, tomorrow or next week. She won't say something to you like, look what you've done to your mouth now because of the things that Dr. Fox will need to treat. These types of comments in the past, now or in the future don't help people to stop the thumb suck habit. Does this sound good to you?"

Susie: "That sounds great."

Dr. Fox: "The first thing I'll do is find out when do you suck? Do you suck in the daytime while you're awake?"

Susie: "Yes."

Mom: "She sucks in the car."

Dr. Fox: "Thank you for your answer, but right now I only want the time and not places the suck occurs. Also, the questions are directed towards Susie so that she and I talk why you listen and we'll get your help if we need to."

Mom: "You're right, I forgot."

Dr. Fox: "Susie let's get back to this. Susie, if you don't mind when we talk please look at me and my eyes. I'm over here. If you ask me how my day was, and I look over the other way, does that look good to you?"

Susie: "No." (Susie then looks at Dr. Fox).

Dr. Fox: "Do you suck your thumb before you lay down to go to sleep?"

Susie: "No."

Dr. Fox: "Do you suck your thumb before you fall asleep after your head lays down on the pillow?"

Susie: "Yes."

Dr. Fox: "Does the thumb stay in your mouth after you fall asleep and stays in the mouth most of the night?"

Suzie: "Yes, I believe so."

Dr. Fox: "Is it in your mouth when you wake up in the morning?"

Susie: "No."

Dr. Fox: "Susie, we basically have four types of thumb suckers. Someone who sucks day and night, daytime only, before bed only and nighttime only. You're a day and night thumb sucker.

Now let's move on to locations where you suck your thumb. We already know that you suck your thumb in your sleep on the bed. Do you suck your thumb when you come home from school and get on the sofa?"

Susie: "Yes."

Dr. Fox: "Do you suck your thumb after you do your homework and you watch television around 7:00 PM?"

Susie: "Yes."

Dr. Fox: "Do you suck your thumb under the bed or in a closet with the door closed?"

Susie: "(Giggles) No, who will do that?"

Dr. Fox: "I want to find all the places that you do this so that later in the hour we can help you not suck in those places. Do you suck your thumb in the backseat of a car on a short trip to the grocery store?"

Susie: "No. But, if I'm in the car more than twenty minutes I'll do it. We just went on a trip last Sunday that was over an hour drive and I did it in the backseat."

Dr. Fox: "Thank you. Do you do it at the movie theater where it's dark and no one can see you?"

Susie: "Yes."

Dr. Fox: "So, it seems like you don't suck your thumb anywhere where there's a chance that someone may see you do it except for others in your family, right?"

Susie: "Yes."

Dr. Fox: "So, is there anything else you want to tell me about times and locations where you suck your thumb?"

Susie: "No (mom is in the background and shakes her head no)."

Dr. Fox: "Which finger or thumb do you suck? Can you point to it?"

Susie: "It's this one." (Suzie holds her right thumb up in the air and points to it with her left index finger).

Dr. Fox: "Do you suck the other thumb or any other fingers?"

Susie: "No."

Dr. Fox: "Do you suck any of your toes?"

Susie: "No. But, I remember that I use to years ago."

Dr. Fox: "Thank you. Are you okay right now? I haven't said anything that bothers you or made you feel bad?"

Susie: "No. I'm fine."

Dr. Fox: "Do you suck on a blanket at night, before bed or in the day?"

Susie: "No. I do sleep with a teddy bear that I've had for years."

Dr. Fox: "All is okay. Do you suck on any pens, other objects or a binky (pacifier)?"

Susie: "No. Mom told me that I used to have a binky, but I don't remember it."

Dr. Fox: "Good. The next thing we do is fun. What this will do is give you the power to stop suck your thumb even though you have had this power to stop before today, but you didn't realize it. Let's start.

First, let's pretend that you go to the mall with three of your friends this Saturday. Do you ever go to the mall?"

Susie: "Yes, all the time."

Dr. Fox: "Now, pretend that you this Saturday will walk around with your three friends and have fun. Can you see this or imagine it?"

Susie: "Yes."

Dr. Fox: "Will you suck your thumb while you do this at the mall with your friends?"

Susie: "No."

Dr. Fox: "Why not?"

Susie: "Because I don't want my friends to see me suck my thumb because they'll think I'm a baby, say bad things to me or make me feel I'm bad."

Dr. Fox: "Good, you made the right decision. Now, let's play a game of pretend. What if you're at the mall with your friends 24 hours straight, you don't need to sleep, and you don't get tired. Will you suck your thumb?"

Susie: "Uh, well (she thinks about it for 10 seconds), no, I won't."

Dr. Fox: "That's interesting, isn't it? So, you do have the ability to not suck your thumb for 24 hours. So, you really do not need to suck your thumb, right?"

Susie: "No." (The child appears to brighten up and her eyebrows lift in amazement).

Dr. Fox: "Susie, now let's go do something else that's fun. I want you to tell me three very important people that you have seen on TV that you'll like to meet. They can be a sports player, a person you saw in a movie or a singer."

Susie: "I can only think of one; it's Lady Gaga." (Child looks at mom).

Mom: "You do like Lady Gaga. But, what about Miley Cyrus and Selena Gomez?"

Susie: "Yes, let's have those three as my answers."

Dr. Fox: "Great. Now, I want you to pick one of these three that you pretend will come over tonight to have dinner, sit at the table beside you to eat and they'll spend the night in your home."

Suzie: "Wow, that will be Selena."

Dr. Fox: "So, imagine she has gotten out of her limousine and walks to the front door; you open it, say hello and talk. You have her come to the dinner table and sit beside you. Will you suck your thumb in front of her?"

Susie: "No way."

Dr. Fox: "Why not?"

Susie: "Because I don't want her to think I'm a baby. I'll get embarrassed."

Dr. Fox: "She'll spend the night, sleep in your bed and your parents will have you sleep on a cot in the same room. Will you suck your thumb while Selena is in your bedroom?"

Susie: "No way."

Dr. Fox: "Imagine this celebrity is with you 24 hours a day, you won't suck your thumb, right?"

Susie: "No. It'll be awesome to be with her 24 hours."

Dr. Fox: "You then have the power to decide to carry that same thought you have right now in your mind every minute of the day and night and decide not to ever suck your thumb again, yes?" (I said this while I moved my head vertically up and down to encourage a yes answer, but I didn't say anything and waited for the child to say yes.)

Susie: "Yes, I can."

Dr. Fox: "Now, let's go do something also fun, but different. Imagine you're in front of your class at school and you tell them about the weekend you had. While you tell them your weekend story, you try to decide whether to put your thumb in your mouth for them to see. You don't because why?"

Susie: "Because they'll laugh at me and think I'm dog meat (means a bad or weird person)."

Dr. Fox: "That's awesome. Imagine these classmates are with you 24 hours a day; you won't suck your thumb, right?"

Susie: "No."

Dr. Fox: "So, you do have the power to decide to carry that same thought in your mind every minute of the day and night and decide not to ever suck your thumb again, right?"

Susie: "Yes."

Dr. Fox: "What's your favorite sport you like to play?"

Suzie: "Softball."

Dr. Fox: "You like to hit the ball?"

Susie: "Yes."

Dr. Fox: "What position do you like to play?"

Susie: "First base."

Dr. Fox: "While you play first base do you suck your thumb?"

Susie: "No."

Dr. Fox: "How about when you sit on the bench while you wait your turn to bat?"

Susie: "No."

Dr. Fox: "Imagine right now that you'll play baseball 24 hours a day, you won't need to sleep, and you won't suck your thumb, true?"

Susie: "Yes."

Dr. Fox: "You do have the ability to decide not to suck your thumb if you think you will play baseball 24 hours a day?"

Susie: "Yes."

Dr. Fox: "Great! We're almost finished with this step. Can you do anything about a problem that occurred last week, last year or two years ago?"

Susie: "No."

Dr. Fox: "Can you do anything about a problem in five minutes from now?"

Susie: "Yes. Because it hasn't happened yet."

Dr. Fox: "Can you do anything about something next week or next year?"

Susie: "Yes."

Dr. Fox: "What's the point to all of this? There's nothing you can do about the past ... only the present and future. Do you agree with this?"

Susie: "Yes. I can only do things now and in the future."

Dr. Fox: "Can you do anything about sucking your thumb this morning, last night, yesterday, last week or last year?"

Susie: "No."

Dr. Fox: "You have the ability to solve a problem that exists now. Right?"

Susie: "Yes."

Dr. Fox: "You also have the right to forgive yourself because of a mistake you made in the past, correct?"

Susie: "Yes."

Dr. Fox: "You have my permission to start fresh, right now and never thumb suck again and pretend that it never happened since it's now only a memory. Is that okay with you?"

Susie: "Yes."

Dr. Fox: "Susie, you made the right decision. Awesome! Again, do you realize you have the power to stop and start anything, control this habit and just let it go forever and never do it ever?"

Susie: "Yes, I have the ability to stop suck my thumb." (This was the key answer I needed from Susie).

Dr. Fox: "Great! Let's go to the next step that will help you help yourself at different places and times to not get in a situation where you feel like you need to suck. We'll handle the urges that pop up day to day and how to make those urges go away. Sound good?"

Susie: "Yes."

Dr. Fox: "We're just about halfway finished. Are you okay? You're not tired or hungry?"

Susie: "No."

Dr. Fox: "Has there been anything that I've said that sounded negative, makes you feel bad or you feel like I said it to make you feel bad?"

Susie: "No."

Dr. Fox: "We'll now go to the next step. We'll go back and forth places that you suck and don't suck your thumb. Tell me where you suck your thumb. Do you do it at home on the sofa when you come home from school a little tired?"

Susie: "Yes."

Dr. Fox: "Have you done it at home on a Sunday afternoon when you're tired or bored with nothing to do?"

Susie: "Yes."

Dr. Fox: "Do you suck your thumb in the back seat of a car on a vacation trip or short trip to the grocery store?"

Susie: "Yes."

Dr. Fox: "Do you suck your thumb at night when you go to bed?"

Susie: "Yes."

Dr. Fox: "Do you suck before you fall asleep to help you go to sleep?"

Susie: "Yes."

Dr. Fox: "Now, let's go into all the places where you don't suck your thumb. Do you do it in front of your class when you're at school?"

Susie: "No."

Dr. Fox: "Do you suck your thumb when you go out to dinner with your parents?"

Susie: "No."

Dr. Fox: "How about in front of your friends at a birthday party; do you suck your thumb?"

Susie: "No."

Dr. Fox: "Do you really need to suck your thumb?"

Susie: "No, I don't need to suck my thumb."

Dr. Fox: "Good, you made the right decision. We're ready to go to the next step to help you not get into situations that will cause you to want to suck your thumb like you have in the past. We basically will break up your routine how you do things at times and locations you previously sucked.

So, the easiest one to start with is when you come home from school; don't sit down and watch television. First, I want your mom to fix you something to eat and drink that won't ruin your dinner.

Not a bunch of sugar either. Bread and sugar will make you sleepy and tired. Have something like celery sticks, vegetables and a piece of chicken that gives energy. Many people like you eat lunch at noon, but don't eat dinner until six or eight o'clock and that's a long time to go without a meal.

After you eat, go outside and do something after you tell your mom. Ride a horse, bike or shoot basketball's, but don't get on that sofa. Why is that?"

Susie: "Because I'll get on the sofa, get bored and suck my thumb."

Dr. Fox: "Great! Rather than go outside you can take karate classes, paint classes or do something that allows you to learn something new you're good at. Some people at your age take golf lessons or learn how to play a simple musical instrument as a guitar. To learn the piano is too complex. I'll talk more later about other ideas I have for you to do after school. Let's go to another situation where you've sucked.

Before sleep, I know that you told me you suck. So, I want you very tired so that you don't need to suck your thumb to fall asleep. What time do you go to sleep?"

Susie: "7:00 PM. I get up at 6:30 AM."

Dr. Fox: "If it's okay with your mom, I want you to stay up until 8 PM."

Mom: "That sounds okay."

Dr. Fox: "Mom, for her age, 7 PM is too early for bed and she gets too much rest. From 7 to 8 PM, I don't want her to lay on the sofa. Try to avoid TV, but if she must, I want her to sit in a chair so that she doesn't get sleepy, lies down and the thumb makes its way into the mouth. This way, she'll be tired when she goes to sleep.

When you go to bed, I want your mom to pull up a chair beside the bed to give you a back massage while you turn away from her so that you'll relax and go to sleep without your thumb. If she sits on your bed and gets up, you'll wake up from her movement. Does that sound good, Susie?"

Susie: "Yes."

Dr. Fox: "Mom, rub her shoulders and back with medium pressure and then as she goes to sleep, use less pressure to barely touch her pajamas. Then, get up and tiptoe out of the room. Please don't check back on her since this will wake her up. Mom, I want you to do this for at least a week.

Now let's go to the next location. The backseat of the car. For the next 30 days, to break up your routine, your mom will sit in the back seat and you sit in the front seat as your dad drives the car. Or, mom will set in the backseat with you as a second choice. Does this sound good, Susie?"

Susie: "Yes."

Dr. Fox: "Susie, realize that I don't want you to put yourself into situations, places or locations that'll make you want to suck your thumb. I realize that you do know what a habit is and that it's something that you don't have to do, but for some reason you do it. Just like people who smoke cigarettes. Do you ever see people smoke cigarettes?"

Susie: "Yes."

Dr. Fox: "Do you ever see people who drink alcohol too much?"

Susie: "Yes."

Dr. Fox: "Do you ever see fat people that eat too much?"

Susie: "Yes."

Dr. Fox: "The point to all of this is that these people need to break up their routine and not put themselves in situations that require them to smoke, drink or eat when they didn't need to. A friend asks a person on a diet who is 100 pounds overweight to go get some ice cream. Is this a good idea?"

Susie: "No. They must go elsewhere that serve salads. Or, go for walk or ride a bicycle."

Dr. Fox: "Very good. We'll now go to the last step. Everything's okay?"

Susie: "Yes."

Dr. Fox: "Do you know what age a baby or infant is?"

Susie: "Up to age four."

Dr. Fox: "Thank you for your answer, but the age is up to age one. Did you know that you mustn't suck your thumb past the age of two?"

Susie: "No."

Dr. Fox: "Do you know that to suck is for babies up to age one?"

Susie: "No."

Dr. Fox: "Raise your right hand and show me how old you are with your fingers."

Susie: "I'm six." (She holds up all four fingers and thumb on the right hand and her index finger on her left hand).

Dr. Fox: "Good. Susie, up to what age are you able to suck your thumb as a baby?"

Susie: "One."

Dr. Fox: "Use your left hand and show me your fingers what your answer is."

Susie: "One." (She holds up one finger with her left hand).

Dr. Fox: "You have told me that you're age six and you're not supposed to suck your thumb past age one and that babies are up to age one. Are you a baby and is it okay to suck your thumb at age six?"

Susie: "No, I'm not a baby and it's not okay to suck my thumb."

Dr. Fox: "Very good answer. Now, we'll switch to something else, but like what we just did. Will it be okay if your mom comes to school with you tomorrow and sit there all day long in those tiny first grade chairs you sit in?"

Susie: "No."

Dr. Fox: "Will it be okay for your dad tomorrow to be dressed up in the same uniform you play soccer in and be on the field with you and the other children?"

Susie: "No."

Dr. Fox: "So, think about your mom in the tiny chair and your dad on the soccer field. That will look weird because they're too old to be doing those things, right?"

Susie: "Yes, it'll look weird. They're too old to do that."

Dr. Fox: "Then, is it okay for you to suck your thumb past age one and to look like a baby?"

Susie: "No."

Dr. Fox: "When someone sees you suck your thumb at age 6, what do you think they think?"

Susie: "They think I'm a baby and it's weird that this age six child sucks their thumb past age one."

Dr. Fox: "Very good answer. So, do you feel it's okay for you to suck your thumb at age six any longer?"

Susie: "No."

Dr. Fox: "Do you want to stop suck your thumb right now and never do it again?"

Susie: "Yes."

Dr. Fox: "Do you know you've hurt your teeth and your teeth don't fit together in the front?"

Susie: "Yes."

Dr. Fox: "Will you take a hammer and hit your big toe on your right foot?"

Susie: "No."

Dr. Fox: "Will you take that same hammer and hit and break your teeth?"

Susie: "No."

Dr. Fox: "Susie, I know you don't use a hammer, but the thumb hurts your teeth and I don't want you to hurt them any longer. Is that okay with you?"

Susie: "Yes."

Dr. Fox: "We're almost finished. Let me help you not hurt your teeth with positive reminders to not put your thumb in your mouth. We'll then set up a reward system to achieve the goal to not suck your thumb for 30 days. Then, we know it's gone. Positive reminders give you protection in the day. Even if you've already done this, we'll use Band-Aids in a different, easy way.

Let me show you how they're placed. I have some here. Place one Band-Aid on the thumb with the cotton portion on the inside part of the thumb away from the nail at the first knuckle. A second Band-Aid is placed over the first one, half way up towards the nail, but be sure neither Band-Aid is too tight. Bend your thumb now to make sure you're able to bend your thumb, yet the Band-Aid won't come off.

Susie: "It's okay." (She bends her thumb).

Dr. Fox: "That looks good. Keep a small baggie with four Band-Aids in it. The Band-Aids must stay on you. If a Band-Aid gets wet or falls off, you must have Band-Aids to put back on. If I or your mom ask you to show us your baggie of Band-Aids and you pull them out of your pocket and show us means that you intend 100% to stop your thumb suck habit.

Change the Band-Aids different times of the day. The skin under the Band-Aid will look wrinkled like a raisin if you leave them on too long. We'll know if you sucked your thumb in the night because your Band-Aids will be wet in the morning.

Go to the store with mom and buy Band-Aids with cartoons on them or you can draw on plain ones with a magic marker. I want you to make this fun. No one will know that you wear Band-Aids for your thumb suck habit. If someone asks, tell them that you have a paper cut.

I have three important rules. First, don't remove the Band-Aids. The Band-Aids aren't punishment, they're only a reminder to not suck your thumb. I won't be happy with you and be disappointed if you remove the Band-Aids to suck.

The second rule is, if you must suck your thumb you must do it with the Band-Aids on. Do you agree?"

Susie: "Yes."

Dr. Fox: "Give me your right hand. Let's shake hands that you'll try 100% not to take the Band-Aids off and that if you must suck you'll suck with the Band-Aids on. (We shook hands in agreement).

The third rule is also important. Have you ever wondered why you only suck your right thumb and not the left one or any of the other eight fingers?"

Susie: "No, you're right. I don't know why."

Dr. Fox: "Well, if you suck your thumb with or without the Band-Aids, you'll also need to suck every finger and the left thumb one minute each. This isn't punishment. The fingers and left thumb get lonely and it's not fair to give all your attention to your right thumb. Give me a handshake that you'll do this rule if you suck your right thumb even if it is with the Band-Aids on."

Susie: "Yes." (She shakes my hand in agreement).

Dr. Fox: "So, let's go over the three rules again. Give me your hand and while we shake hands you'll agree that you won't remove the Band-Aids, you'll suck your thumb if you must with the Band-Aids on and that you'll also suck all other eight fingers and left thumb for one minute each if you suck your thumb."

Susie: "Yes." (She shakes my hand in agreement).

Dr. Fox: "The last thing to do is set up a reward system because everything in life is about goals and things we want to have or achieve. Goals and achievements need rewarded once reached. It's easier to achieve goals if we break each goal into smaller steps and reward each step along the way.

You mustn't suck your thumb for thirty days or four weeks. At the end of each week a reward needs to be decided between you and your mom.

It's best to discuss this on the way home with your mom; I bet she already has some ideas. I don't want you to push mom for something you want, but the two of you can talk and figure out what the reward will be. Don't change your mind every day what each reward will be; set these weekly goals and rewards and stick to your decisions. Then, when you've reached 30 days in a row of no thumb suck you'll get your final reward.

Keep a calendar on the refrigerator that has squares for each day. Each morning, put a check or an S in the square for the previous day and night. If you touched your thumb to your mouth even for a second that's an S and you must start the 30 days again. Yes, it'll frustrate you when this happens.

The first week reward can be a small item especially if it's something you want to get anyway. If you must get clothes for school, I understand. But, try not to buy anything for the next 30 days except these weekly rewards. No, I don't expect your mom to buy you a horse or car as your final reward. This is totally between you and her; not me.

Mom, I want you to keep her busy. In addition to her homework, find something creative. Play video games and be on the phone isn't creative. Take an art class. It doesn't cost much money to go to the art store and buy charcoal pencils and paper. Have her draw things that are in front of her like a house or something she sees on the Internet. Draw it perfectly as it is. One of my six-year-old patients drew horses and later in life decided to be an artist.

Search on the Internet for a guitar and lessons under $100 from a guitar teacher Estabon. Do golf lessons. She must create things in the physical, real-world and not something in her mind.

Most thumb suckers are very bored, don't create enough and are very smart. We must get her to use her mind and abilities. You'll find something she loves to do, is very passionate about and maybe her next career. Tiger Woods swung his first golf club at age 2."

Susie: "We're finished. I want you to call me in 24 hours to personally let me know that you didn't suck your thumb and that you feel it has stopped. Also, I want to talk to you in 4 to 6 days in person for a quick fifteen minutes and we need to set that time up now. I'm very proud of you right now to make this decision to stop and that you'll get 30 checkmarks in a row on your calendar. Then, we'll know this thumb suck habit is totally gone forever. I'm very proud of you. Good luck!

CHAPTER 17

Sample: Begin to End Treatment of a First Session Adult Thumb Sucker

Present in the room today is Jack and his wife. Jack's thirty-one years old and began a new job last week as an accountant for a CPA firm. Jack sits in a chair and faces me about three feet apart. His wife, Karen, has been told to only answer questions that are directed at her and not to help her husband. The wife sits behind and to the left of the husband so that the husband can turn and see her if he needs to.

The back of the throat has been checked four weeks ago and there were large tonsils and adenoids associated with breathing problems and dark rings under the eyes. He woke up six times a night with a dry mouth and his wife indicated he snored severe that kept her up to the point where she had to sleep in another bedroom. I referred him to have the tonsils and adenoids removed. Afterwards, he stated it was a quality of life change for him. He now has more energy around 4 PM each day and sleeps most of the night only to wake to urinate. His wife now sleeps in the same bed.

There are no home problems. He had a medical physical three months ago and didn't take psychiatric medications.

I made sure he ate protein food with no sugar since it was 5 o'clock in the afternoon and he wasn't tired. You don't want to do these techniques in this book if the patient is hungry, sleepy or had a rough day. Reschedule if everything isn't perfect.

Dr. Fox: "Jack, I'm here to discuss with you about your thumb suck habit. You do realize you have one, right?"

Jack: "Yes, I'm very embarrassed about all of this."

Dr. Fox: "Look at the pictures in the front of this book and see these people suck on different things. What does this picture look like?"

Jack: "A baby."

Dr. Fox: "Great. (Continued to show 4 more photos with the same answers). Now, here are some photos that show you do the same. What does this photo look like?"

Jack: "A baby."

Dr. Fox: "Very good. I've shown you these photos to help you realize that you need to see yourself with this habit because many times I find a person with this habit only sees things through their eyes and not from a distance. Many times, a thumb sucker doesn't see themselves do this habit as if they were to do a selfie photo or video while they suck.

Put all the things that seem negative to you not in your thoughts anymore. I really believe if you want to stop you will and that's why you want me to help you. Do you want to stop?"

Jack: "Yes."

Dr. Fox: "Everything we're about to do is only positive over the next half an hour to one hour. If anything I say to you sounds negative or makes you feel bad, raise your right hand

and I'll stop immediately and ask you what I said that's negative.

From this point onward, your wife will keep all negative off you. This includes comments as look what you've done to your mouth. These comments don't stop the thumb suck habit. Does this sound good to you?"

Jack: "Yes."

Dr. Fox: "The first thing we'll do is to find out when you suck? Do you suck in the daytime while you're awake?"

Jack: "No."

Dr. Fox: "Do you suck your thumb before you lay down to go to sleep?"

Jack: "Yes."

Dr. Fox: "Do you suck your thumb before you fall asleep after your head lays down on the pillow?"

Jack: "Yes."

Dr. Fox: "Does the thumb stay in your mouth after you fall asleep and stays in the mouth most of the night?"

Jack: "Yes."

Dr. Fox: "Is it in your mouth when you wake up in the morning?"

Jack: "Yes."

Dr. Fox: "Jack, we basically have four types of thumb suckers. Someone who sucks day and night, daytime only, before bed only and nighttime only. You're a night thumb sucker.

Now let's move on to locations where you suck your thumb. We already know that you suck your thumb in your sleep on the bed. Do you suck your thumb when you come home from work when you get on the sofa?"

Jack: "No."

Dr. Fox: "Do you suck your thumb when you watch television around 7:00 PM?"

Jack: "No. I'm curious why you ask about sucking different places in the day because I don't do it in the day?"

Dr. Fox: "Very good question. Please don't hesitate to ask me anything because I'm here to help you. The reason is because some people fall asleep in the day and suck and I need to make sure I uncover everywhere and every time you do it. Do you suck your thumb under the bed or in a closet with the door closed?"

Jack: "No, but I used to go in the upstairs entrance to the attic and do it until I was 15 years old."

Dr. Fox: "Do you do it at the movie theater where it's dark and no one can see you?"

Jack: "No."

Dr. Fox: "So, it seems like you don't suck your thumb anywhere where there's a chance that someone may see you do it except for others in your family, right?"

Jack: "Yes."

Dr. Fox: "So, is there anything else you want to tell me about time and locations where you suck your thumb?"

Jack: "No."

Dr. Fox: "Which finger or thumb do you suck? Can you point to it?"

Jack: Jack holds his left thumb up in the air.

Dr. Fox: "Do you suck the other thumb or any other fingers?"

Jack: "No."

Dr. Fox: "The next question I ask will sound odd and I don't want to offend you, but I must be very thorough. Do you suck any of your toes?"

Jack: "No."

Dr. Fox: "Thank you. Are you okay right now? I haven't said anything that bothers you or made you feel bad?"

Jack: "No. I'm okay."

Dr. Fox: "Do you suck on a blanket in the night, before bed or in the day?"

Jack: "No. I used to walk around with a blanket all the time like Linus on Charlie Brown until the age of six."

Dr. Fox: "All is okay. Do you suck on any pens, other objects or a binky (pacifier)?"

Jack: "No."

Dr. Fox: "Good. The next thing we'll do is fun. What this will do is give you the power to stop thumb suck even though you have had this power to stop before today, but didn't realize it. Let's start.

First, let's pretend that you'll go to the football game with three of your friends this Sunday. You walk around with your three friends and you'll have fun. Can you see this or imagine it?"

Jack: "Yes."

Dr. Fox: "Are you sucking your thumb while you do this at the football stadium with your friends?"

Jack: "No."

Dr. Fox: "Why not?"

Jack: "Because they'll think I'm a baby and think less of me."

Dr. Fox: "Excellent. Now, let's play a game of pretend. What if you are at a football game with your friends 24 hours straight and you won't need to sleep, won't get tired and everyone has fun. Will you suck your thumb?"

Jack: "No, I won't."

Dr. Fox: "That's awesome, isn't it? So, you do have the ability to not suck your thumb for 24 hours, right?"

Jack: "Yes."

Dr. Fox: "Jack, now let's go to something else that's fun. Tell me three very important people that you've seen on TV that you'll like to meet. They can be a sports player, actor or singer."

Jack: "I can only think of one and its Peyton Manning, retired quarterback. And, Bill Gates owner of Microsoft and Simon who used to be on American Idol."

Dr. Fox: "Great. Now, I want you to pick one of the three that we'll pretend will come over tonight, sit at the table beside you at dinner and they'll also spend the night in your home."

Jack: "Wow, that'll have to be Bill Gates."

Dr. Fox: "So, imagine he has gotten out of his limousine, walks to the front door and you open it, say hello and talk. You have him come to the dinner table and sit beside you. Will you suck your thumb in front of Bill Gates?"

Jack: "No."

Dr. Fox: "Why not?"

Jack: "Because I don't want to get embarrassed."

Dr. Fox: "He'll spend the night and sleep in your bed and you'll have to sleep in another bedroom or sofa. Will you suck your thumb while he's in your bedroom?"

Jack: "No."

Dr. Fox: "If this celebrity is with you 24 hours a day, you won't suck your thumb, right?"

Jack: "No. It'll be awesome to be with him 24 hours."

Dr. Fox: "You then have the power to decide to carry this same thought in your mind every minute of the day and night and decide not to ever suck your thumb again?" (I said this while I moved my head vertically up and down to encourage a yes answer, but I don't say anything and wait for Jack to say yes.)

Jack: "Yes, I can."

Dr. Fox: "Now, let's go on to something also fun, but different. Imagine you're in front of your accountants at a work meeting and you tell them about an idea you have. While you tell them, you try to decide whether to put your thumb in your mouth for them to see. You don't because why?"

Jack: "Because they'll fire me."

Dr. Fox: "Okay. If these fellow workers are with you 24 hours a day you won't suck your thumb, right?"

Jack: "No."

Dr. Fox: "So, you do have the power to decide not to ever suck your thumb again, right?"

Jack: "Yes."

Dr. Fox: "What's your favorite sport you like to play?"

Jack: "Tennis."

Dr. Fox: "While you play tennis do you suck your thumb?"

Jack: "No."

Dr. Fox: "How about when you sit on the bench while you rest between sets?"

Jack: "No."

Dr. Fox: "Pretend you'll play tennis 24 hours a day if you won't have to sleep?"

Jack: "Yes, I can pretend that since I love tennis."

Dr. Fox: "You do have the ability to decide not to suck your thumb if you think you'll play tennis 24 hours a day?"

Jack: "Yes."

Dr. Fox: "Great! Were almost finished with this step. Can you do anything about last week, last year or two years ago?"

Jack: "No."

Dr. Fox: "Can you do anything about something in five minutes from now?"

Jack: "Yes. Because it hasn't happened yet."

Dr. Fox: "Can you do anything about something next week or next year?"

Jack: "Yes."

Dr. Fox: "What is the point to all of this? There's nothing you can do about the past ... only the present and future. Do you agree with this?"

Jack: "Yes."

Dr. Fox: "Can you do anything about sucking your thumb this last night, yesterday, last week or last year?"

Jack: "No."

Dr. Fox: "You have the ability to solve a problem that exists now. Right?"

Jack: "Yes."

Dr. Fox: "You can also forgive yourself for a mistake you made in the past. Right?"

Jack: "Yes."

Dr. Fox: "You have my permission to start fresh, right now and never thumb suck again and pretend that it never happened since it's now only a memory. Is that okay with you?"

Jack: "Yes."

Dr. Fox: "Jack, you made the right decision. Great! Realize that you have the power to stop, start and control this habit. Just let it go forever and never do it again?"

Jack: "Yes, I really do see that I can stop my thumb suck habit." (This was the key answer I needed from Jack).

Dr. Fox: "Great! Let's move on to the next step to help you in different places and times so you can help yourself not get in the situation where you feel like you need to suck. We'll handle the urges that pop up day to day and how to make those urges go away. Sound good?"

Jack: "Yes."

Dr. Fox: "We're about half way finished. Are you okay? You're not tired or hungry?"

Jack: "No. I'm fine."

Dr. Fox: "Has there been anything that I've said that sounded negative or makes you feel bad?"

Jack: "No."

Dr. Fox: "We'll now go to the next step. If possible, we'll talk later more about this next thing, but try some new creative things like karate or paint classes to take your mind off the urge to suck. Learn something new you're good at. Take golf lessons or learn how to play a simple musical instrument as a guitar. We'll come back to this later.

Before sleep, I know that you told me you suck. So, what I want you to do is be very tired when you go to sleep so that you don't have to suck your thumb. What time do you go to sleep?"

Jack: "10:00 PM. I get up at 7:30 AM."

Dr. Fox: "If it's okay with you, I want you to stay up until 11 PM."

Jack: "Yes."

Dr. Fox: "From 8 until 11 PM don't lie on the sofa to watch TV because I don't want you to prematurely fall asleep. This way, you'll be tired when you go to sleep.

The next thing I want is your wife will pull up a chair beside your bed. I don't want her to get on the bed because she'll give you a back massage while you turn away from her so that you can relax and go to sleep without your thumb. If she sets on your bed and gets up, she'll wake you. Does that sound good to you, Jack?"

Jack: "Yes."

Dr. Fox: "Karen, rub his shoulders and back with medium pressure and after he's gone to sleep barely touch his pajamas. Then, get up and tiptoe out of the room or go to the other side of the bed and get in the bed quietly. Karen, I want you to do this for at least a week.

Around 9:30 PM you can have a cup of Sleepy Time Tea that's decaffeinated. Don't drink coffee or cocoa. Refrain from sugar after 9:00 PM. Take a walk will be helpful.

Now, let's change to important information about the thumb suck habit that you may have or haven't thought about. Do you know what age a baby or infant is?"

Jack: "Up to age two."

Dr. Fox: "The age is only up to age one. Did you know that you don't suck your thumb past age two?"

Jack: "Yes."

Dr. Fox: "Do you know that sucking is for babies up to age one?"

Jack: "No."

Dr. Fox: "How old are you?"

Jack: "I'm thirty-one."

Dr. Fox: "Good. Jack, up to what age are you able to suck your thumb as a baby?"

Jack: "One."

Dr. Fox: "You've told me that you are age thirty-one and you're not to suck your thumb past age two and that babies are up to age one. Are you a baby and is it okay to suck at age thirty-one?"

Jack: "No, I'm not a baby and it's not okay to suck my thumb."

Dr. Fox: "Very good answer. Do you know you've hurt your teeth and that your teeth don't fit together in the front?"

Jack: "Yes."

Dr. Fox: "You won't take a hammer and hit your big toe on your foot, will you?"

Jack: "No."

Dr. Fox: "You won't take that same hammer and hit your teeth and break them?"

Jack: "No."

Dr. Fox: "Jack, you didn't use a hammer, but the thumb hurt your teeth and we don't want you to hurt them anymore. Is that okay with you?"

Jack: "Yes."

Dr. Fox: "I'll help you with this. We're almost finished, but we need to go into some positive reminders to help you not put your thumb in your mouth before bed. We'll then set up a reward system to help you not suck your thumb for thirty days and then we'll know it's gone. Let's first get into the positive reminders to help give you protection. You may have already done this, but we'll use Band-Aids.

But, the Band-Aids are placed on your thumb a certain way. Let me show you how they are placed on; I have some here. Go to the store and get Band-Aids with cartoons on them or you can draw on plain Band-Aids with a magic marker. I want you to make this fun. No one will know that you do this because of your thumb suck habit.

Place one Band-Aid on the thumb with the cotton portion on the inside part of the thumb away from the nail at the first knuckle. A second Band-Aid is placed over the first one half way up towards the nail, but be sure neither Band-Aid is too tight. Make sure you're still able to bend your thumb, yet the Band-Aid won't come off."

Jack: (he bends his thumb).

Dr. Fox: "That looks good. Keep a small baggie with six Band-Aids in it. I want you to put the Band-Aids on at 8:00 PM so that you're used to them when you go to sleep at 11:00 PM. That lets me know you want to try 100%.

Interestingly, we'll know if you suck your thumb in the night because your Band-Aids will be wet in the morning.

I do have one more rule and it's the most important rule. These Band-Aids aren't punishment, they're only a reminder to stop suck your thumb. I won't be happy with you and I'll become very disappointed if you remove the Band-Aids and then suck your thumb. If you must suck your thumb you must do it with the Band-Aids on. Do you agree?"

Jack: "Yes."

Dr. Fox: "Give me your right hand. Shake hands that you'll try 100% to not take the Band-Aids off. (I shook hands in agreement with Jack). The next rule's also important. Have you ever wondered why you only suck your right thumb and not the left one; and the other fingers?"

Jack: "No."

Dr. Fox: "Well, if you suck your thumb with or without the Band-Aids, you'll also need to suck every other finger and thumb one minute each. This isn't punishment. It's not fair to give all your attention to your right thumb. Give me a handshake that you'll do this rule if you suck your thumb even if it's with the Band-Aids on."

Jack: "Yes." (He shakes my hand in agreement).

Dr. Fox: "So, let's go over the three rules again. Give me your hand and while we shake hands you'll agree that you won't remove the Band-Aids, suck your thumb with the Band-Aid on and you'll also suck all other eight fingers and left thumb for one minute each if you suck your thumb."

Jack: "Yes." (He shakes my hand in agreement).

Dr. Fox: "The last thing is to set up a reward system because everything in life is about goals and we need to have goals rewarded once they've been achieved. It's easier to achieve goals if we break them down into little steps and reward each step along the way. You need to stop your thumb suck habit for 30 days or four weeks. At the end of each week a reward needs decided by you.

You'll keep a calendar on the refrigerator that has squares. Put a check or an S in the square in the morning for the previous day and night. If you touch your thumb to your mouth even for a second that's an S and you'll have to start the 30 days over again. Yes, it'll frustrate you. The first week prize or award can be a small item especially if it's something you'll get anyway.

Karen, I want you to keep him busy. I want him to do home projects, but I also want him to start something that's creative. Play video games and be on the phone isn't creative. Take an art class or learn to play a guitar.

Go on the Internet and order a guitar and lessons for under $100 from a guitar teacher Esteban. He can do golf lessons. Anything that he creates he sees in the real physical world and not something in his mind.

Most thumb suckers are very bored, smart and don't create enough. We must get him to use his mind, abilities and you'll find something he loves to do and is very passionate about. It will turn out to be his new hobby and possible career."

Jack: "We're finished. I want one last handshake that you agree 100% not to take the Band-Aids off, you'll only suck with the Band-Aids on and you'll also suck each of the eight fingers and the other thumb one minute each if you suck.

I want you to call me in 24 hours and personally let me know that you didn't suck your thumb and you feel it has stopped. (He shakes my hand). Also, I want to talk to you in four to six days in person for a quick fifteen minutes and we need to set that time up now. I'm very proud of you right now for your decision to stop and that you'll get thirty checkmarks in a row on your calendar. Then, we'll know your thumb suck habit has totally gone. I'm very proud of you. Good luck!"

CHAPTER 18

Age Seven Repair of the Damage from Thumb, Finger, Toe, Pacifier and Blanket Sucking

Dentofacial Orthopedics – The scientific field Thumb Suck treatment is classified under

"To know how to repair the damage to the human body, one must know how the damage occurred in the first place." My favorite quote I invented while I researched how Tylenol causes birth defects and other damage to the body years ago. Many physicians and dentists treat their patients, but don't understand the cause of the patient's problems.

This is called etiology. When you know the etiology of a problem or cause of a problem you'll have a better success to treat the problem and for it not to return. 346 patients never returned to any habit I stopped.

At age seven, to repair the damage from thumb suck, use of a pacifier or blanket suck, the treatment deals with early orthodontic treatment rather than the traditional teenage orthodontic treatment with braces. This treatment at age deals with what we call "orthopedics." Orthopedics is skeletal correction via growth alteration. I have a Master's of Science degree in Orthodontics and Dentofacial Orthopedics.

When I see a child, and notice the damage to their teeth and bone structures, I don't ask questions any longer to the parent or child how they suck because I can tell from the damage that was done. In other locations of this book, the different types of positions of the thumb or finger determines the damage. I don't expect the reader of this book to know the positions of the thumb or finger that caused the damage. But, realize that an expert, as myself with over twenty-five years' experience must be consulted and treatment commenced.

Type 1: Distinguish cause of the open bite from the upper front teeth pushed out by the thumb or the upper back teeth and bone extrude that prevents the upper & lower front teeth to touch.

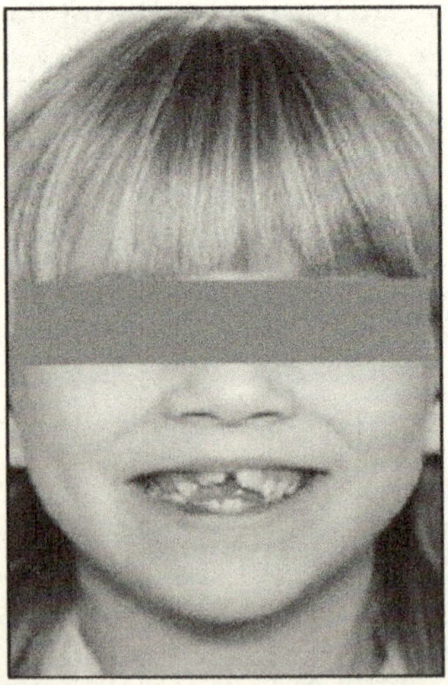

The patient must be diagnosed properly to see if the upper front teeth have been pushed up and out or whether the back upper teeth and bone have extruded. In the situation with upper jaw extrusion, the lower jaw now can't close all the way up and forward. This is due from the "wedge-type" effect caused by the upper back teeth and bone extruded that props the bite open.

If the upper front teeth were pushed up and out, the thumb was placed behind the upper front teeth with little sucking done. I call this hook effect from the thumb bent into a shape of a fish hook and then hooked behind the upper front teeth to push them outward.

If the open bite exists without the upper front teeth tipped forward, the thumb sucker sucked with intensity as they kept the front teeth apart while they sucked the upper back teeth and bone down towards the tongue. This happened because the upper back teeth didn't touch the lower back teeth while the thumb was sucked in the front of the mouth.

Can you tell the difference in the below two photos of two different patients?

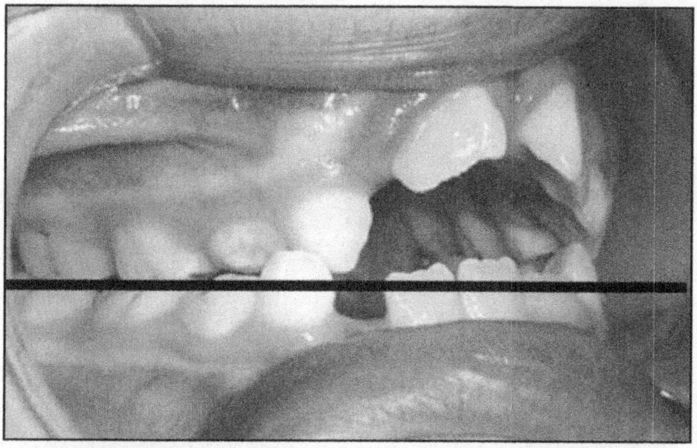

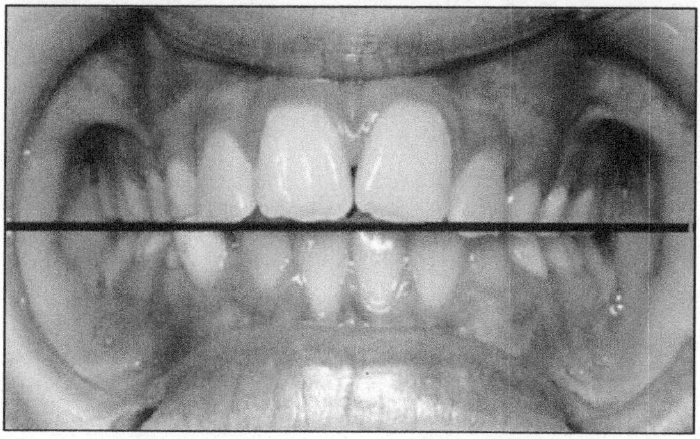

Type 2: The thumb sucker with skinny (narrow) arches.

Look at the thumb sucker straight on as their eyes look at you. Have them smile. If it appears that their teeth aren't wide across or the smile is not broad, but skinny, the thumb sucker used the buccinator muscle (The muscle that goes inward on each cheek when one sucks on a milkshake straw) to push the upper arch inward. The teeth collapsed around the thumb that caused narrow upper and lower arches. Notice the before & after same patient below:

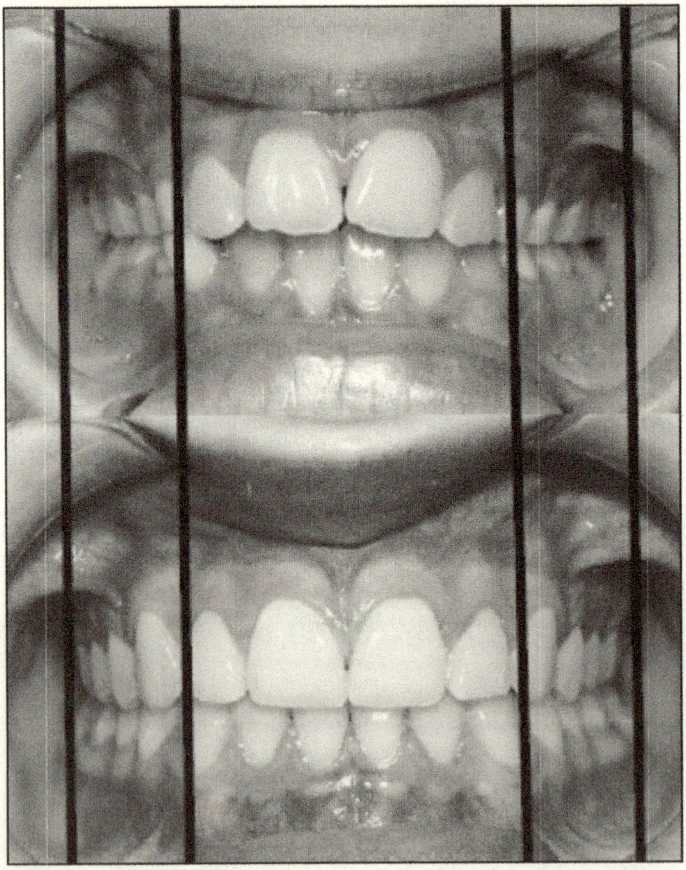

Type 3: Damage to the lower jaw.

The thumb causes the lower jaw to not grow out fully. This is seen in thumb suckers that place their thumb in their mouth pointed up towards their nose instead placed the thumb pointed to the back of their throat. Stop the thumb suck habit won't allow the retruded jaw to grow out to its normal position fully. The damage is permanent unless early interceptive growth treatment begins at age six.

As the thumb sucker gets closer to age ten, the success percentage to get the lower jaw to grow out decreases to less than 30% chance. Between the age of ten and thirteen it is hit and miss whether any jaw growth correction can be achieved and never should be promised.

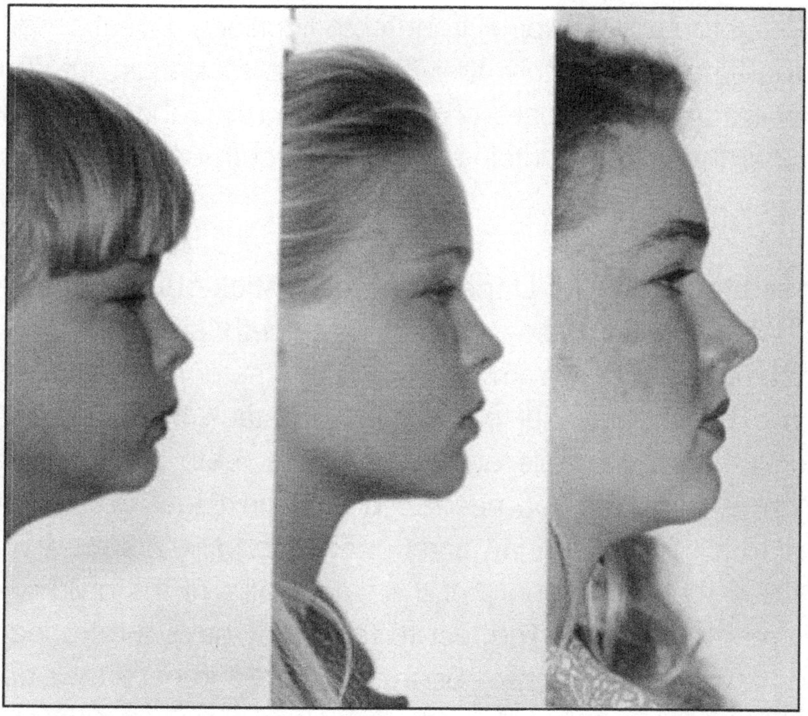

Test: How to tell if the child needs lower jaw growth treatment by an expert Orthodontist highly trained in Dentofacial Orthopedics:

Severe type child: Upper front teeth stick out severe.

Place the seven-year-old child in the chair. Have them sit straight up. They have a severe overjet (upper front teeth stick out from the lower front teeth). You ask yourself, "Should I take the child now to the orthodontist highly trained in age 6 early treatment?" The answer is always yes because an overjet is always classic for jaw growth problems.

Minimally, if the lower jaw isn't retruded (back in position), the upper front teeth must have early teenager braces glued to them and push them in with the braces to prevent the child from fracture of the upper front teeth (incisors). I treat children all the time that fracture their front teeth that stick out. They get hit from sports balls or someone pushes them from the back at the water fountain and hit their teeth on the stainless-steel faucet.

Moderate type child: Upper front teeth stick out moderately.

What if your child's upper front teeth stick out only a moderate amount, 4 mm. or less? A millimeter is the thickness of a dime. If you take four dimes and stack them on top of each other on a table and your child's teeth stick out that much or less then you need to do the next test because it's hard to tell if the lower jaw is retruded (short and not grow out).

See the above photo of the side profile of the child while you read the below. The test to tell if they have a retruded or short lower jaw is simple. Sit the child up and have their back away from the chair. Have them look at a point on the wall. Look at their chin area from the side. If the crease under the lower lip doesn't stick out as far as their forehead point right above their eyebrows, there's a problem.

Notice the above photo of the crease below the lower lip at age seven is further back than the forehead. More importantly, notice the lower lip severely back compared to the upper lip. The left photo is the thumb sucker before any treatment began. The middle photo is after the first expansion step and after the appliance was placed in the roof of the mouth called a transpalatal arch (discussed later in this chapter). The right photo is after lower jaw growth was achieved, braces then placed and removed.

Another test is to have the child hold their incisors end-to-end and look at their profile from the side. If their profile now looks better, you have a lower retruded jaw on your hands. On the other hand, if they now look like Jay Leno with a lower protruded jaw or Abraham Lincoln, the problem is limited to their teeth and lower jaw growth isn't indicated.

Mild type child: No upper front teeth stick out

What if your child has no overjet (the upper teeth don't stick out far from the lower teeth). But, the child seems to have a retruded lower jaw profile or a "no chin" appearance. What usually happens with this type of child is that there's a retruded lower jaw. But, all the lower teeth have shifted forward on the lower arch of bone that gives a "fake Class I normal bite" appearance.

There are three types of bites: Class I normal bite, Class 2 upper teeth stick out bite (which is the above patient photo) and the Class 3 bulldog bite.

Treatment at age seven to repair the damage from thumb suck, pacifier usage or blanket suck:

The three steps of age seven treatment are:

1. Widen the mouth.
2. Open bite closure.
3. Lower jaw growth.

First step of treatment: Widen the mouth.

The first step is to widen the narrow arches with expansion therapy. If moderate to severe crowding exists, serial extractions may also be needed which is selected primary (baby) teeth extracted at different times with eventually four permanent teeth on the sides in the middle of the mouth.

To make the arches wider, I use removable expansion retainers. They look like old fashion retainers used on orthodontic patients after their braces were removed before the year 2000. They're more acceptable than fixed expanders glued to the back molars.

Many fixed or glued-in expanders expand the arches too fast and not allow the cells to break down bone in some areas and other cells to make bone where it's needed. Both removable and fixed expanders must be worn the same amount of time (five to six months). The fixed expanders are expanded quickly and then left in place for four months or more. If both are worn the same amount of time, it's best to expand over the entire time with a removable.

Fixed expanders:

1. Are more expensive because they require a lab to fabricate them.
2. They hurt more because they expand faster with more force.
3. They're uncomfortable because when you turn the expander the force can be felt by the patient and it's

hard to eat with them because they're not removable. This alters the taste of food and the quality of chewing.

4. They're used only in patients that require jaw surgery to expand the bone structures after the age of fifteen. Also, they're used when children are uncooperative with the removable ones.

The above fixed or glued-in expanders data is supported in a journal article, Corbett, Maurice C., Slow and Continuous Maxillary Expansion, Molar Rotation, and Molar Distalization, J. Clin. Orthod. April 1997(253-263). It's been over twenty years, yet the dental profession still violates what I've found to be true in this journal article: The use of these overly forceful, fixed expanders that have a jackscrew glued into the roof of the mouth.

Dr. Corbett's article and references are reprinted below from the Journal of Clinical Orthodontics to emphasize the importance for children to use other expanders that aren't as forceful, but to try to use removable expanders.

Slow and Continuous Maxillary Expansion, Molar Rotation, and Molar Distalization

MAURICE C. CORBETT, DDS

An estimated 25-30% of all orthodontic patients can benefit from maxillary expansion, and 95% of Class II cases can be improved by molar rotation, distalization, and expansion. Rapid palatal expanders such as the Haas and the Hyrax have traditionally been used for treating transverse maxillary discrepancies, but these appliances will not rotate or distalize molars.

Furthermore, rapid palatal expansion has been shown to produce forces ranging from 3 to more than 20 pounds. Studies have documented free-floating bone fragments, bleeding, microfractures, cyst formation, vascular disorganization, and connective tissue inflammation in suture sites during rapid expansion.

Story and Ekstrom have suggested that slow expansion procedures allow physiologic adjustments and reconstitution of the sutural elements over a period of about 30 days. McAndrews demonstrated that the application of light, continuous forces in areas of periosteal growth allows normal arch dimensions to develop at any age without undue tipping of the abutment teeth. Increased fibroblastic, osteoclastic, and osteoblastic activity seems to occur when the maxilla is widened slowly. Slower expansion has also been associated with more physiologic stability and less potential for relapse than with rapid expansion. The neuromuscular adaption of the mandible to the maxilla in slow expansion allows a normal vertical closure.

References

1. McNamara; J.A. Jr. and Brudon, W.L.: *Orthodontic and Orthopedic Treatment in the Mixed Dentition,* Needham Press, Ann Arbor, MI, 1995.
2. Ten Hoeve, A.: Palatal bar and lip bumper in non-extraction treatment, J. Clin. Orthod. 19:272-291, 1985
3. Haas, AJ.: Rapid expansion of the maxillary dental arch and nasal cavity by opening the mid-palatal suture, Angle Orthod.31:73-90,1961.
4. Haas, AJ.: The treatment of maxillary deficiency by opening the mid-palatal suture, Angle Orthod. 35:200-217, 1965.
5. Haas, AJ. Palatal expansion: Just the beginning of dentofacial orthopedics, Am. J. Orthod. 57:219-255, 1970.
6. Bishara, S.E. and Stanley, R.N.: Maxillary expansion Clinical implications, Am. J. Orthod. 91:3-14,198.
7. Hicks, E.P.: Slow maxillary expansion: A clinical study of the skeletal vs. dental response to low magnitude force, Am. J. Orthod. 73:121-141, 1978.
8. Story, E.: Tissue response to the movement of bones, Am. J. Orthod. 64:229-247, 1973.
9. Ekstrom, e.; Henrikson, e.O.; and Jensen, R.: Mineralization in the midpalatal suture after orthodontic expansion, Am. J. Orthod. 71:449-455,1977.
10. McAndrew, J.R.: The continuous force control system, Lancer Technical Report, Lancer Pacific, Carlsbad, CA, 1985.
11. Henry, RJ.: Slow maxillary expansion: A review of quad-helix therapy during the transitional dentition, J. Dent. Child., November-December 1993, pp. 408-413.

12. Bell, R.A. and LeCompte, EJ.: The effects of maxillary expansion using a quad-helix appliance during the deciduous and mixed dentition, Am. J. Orthod. 79:152-161, 1981.
13. Bell, R.A.: A review of maxillary expansion in relation to rate of expansion and patient's age, Am. J. Orthod. 81:32-37,1982.
14. Corbett, M.C.: Molar rotation and beyond, J. Clin. Orthod. 30:272-275, 1996.
15. McConnell, T.L. et al.: Maxillary canine impaction in patients with transverse maxillary deficiency, J. Dent. Child., May-June 1996, pp. 190-195.

A few parents won't listen about removable expanders and will want you to use fixed expanders, but twenty-nine out of thirty children do very well with removable expanders.

Over 80% of the thumb suckers' damage I've treated, closes the open bite at least 50% or more from the expansion step alone.

Second step of treatment: Open bite closure

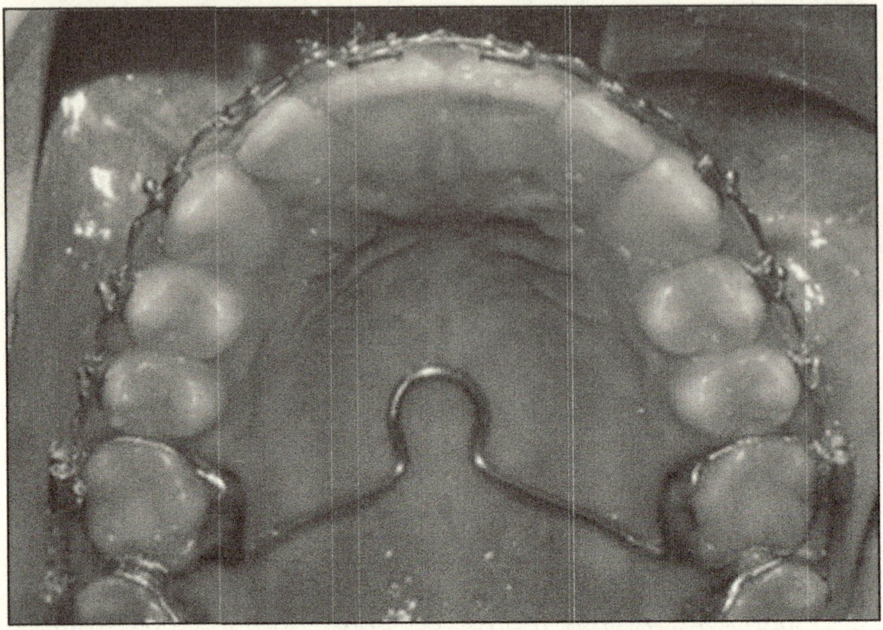

The second step, after the first step of expansion, is to place a special appliance in the roof of the mouth. This is a U-shaped wire that hooks to both upper first molars and runs across the roof of the mouth. This design causes the tongue to hit the wire which makes the upper first molars intrude (direction towards the top of the head).

I tell the thumb sucker that humans swallow 1,500 or more times per day. The normal swallow act has the tongue thrust upward towards the roof of the mouth. We want this device to be in the roof of the mouth so that the tongue hits it 1,500 or more times per day. This causes the intrusion of the upper back molars which are the six back teeth on the upper right and left.

The device is called a Transpalatal Arch. I tell parents and the children that the word "trans" means across just like an airplane flight across the Atlantic is called a transatlantic flight. And the word "palate" is the roof of the mouth. So transpalatal means across the roof of the mouth.

When this appliance is placed, small plastic wedges are made to place between the back molars on the right and left and the patient is asked to clinch on these wedges fifty times every hour. It's important that both sides are done at the same time to not get an uneven bite in the back teeth.

These wedges can be purchased from a dental supplier or find plastic from different things around the house will suffice. Caution needs to be given to not have the child swallow the plastic especially when the plastic starts to wear out or gets smaller.

The wedges must be kept away from animals, especially dogs. If the wedges are laid down anywhere in the house, the dog will chew them as a chew toy into fifty pieces. They'll choke on them to cause the dog to visit a veterinarian on an emergency basis.

Note: There's a treatment step between steps two and three for age seven, severe open bite cases, but it isn't discussed here. It's for advanced training by myself with doctors only in a future book that's in the works now.

Third step of treatment: Lower jaw growth (if needed).

Not all thumb suck damage requires lower jaw growth. Again, it depends on the intensity and position of the thumb, but some patients lower jaw doesn't grow forward due to genetics passed down the genetic tree. In other words, the parents or grandparents may have had this problem and wasn't due to the thumb suck habit.

There are many ways to get the lower jaw to grow forward. Many of the techniques I've personally tried in the past twenty-five years don't truly get the lower jaw to grow forward and only give an appearance that it did.

I have many parents with a twelve-year-old child in the chair tell me how great of an early treatment result their child received from another orthodontist. Mysteriously, as I look at the child, I don't see a great lower jaw profile. I look a little closer and spot that the lower jaw doesn't stick out as far as the forehead or the skin between the upper lip and nose.

I ask the child to hold the lower teeth forward until the lower jaw is the correct position while the upper and lower teeth touch in the back. I tell the child to close their lips gently and the profile now looks perfect and I confirm this with the parent(s). I then hold the lower lip down and out to show that the teeth are now in a bulldog bite. I don't need a lateral cephalometric x-ray (taken of the whole head from the side) that we take for braces to tell me that the lower front teeth are tipped severely forward and the lower jaw growth wasn't achieved by the early treatment.

Contrary to what early treatment research has shown, I do achieve lower jaw growth of the mandible with certain appliances. I do other myofunctional procedures (jaw muscle exercises) along with the appliance that others don't and have found this successful. The past research that stated lower jaw growth is questionable utilized treatments that I know don't work before they even did the research. I know because I tried them.

The age I start treatment is earlier than recent research has shown, yet I do get 90% or higher results. I don't like the appliances worn at the middle school age where the children's hormones and other factors seem to weigh-in to make the child not cooperate.

I've also noticed a 50% or less success rate the closer the child is to age ten. If jaw growth is attempted after the age of ten I'll still try to use certain appliances and if not, resort to full braces and other jaw growth appliances.

Notice the before and after of the same patient below. Notice not only the position of the lower jaw point in reference to the forehead, but the lower lip in reference to the upper lip position.

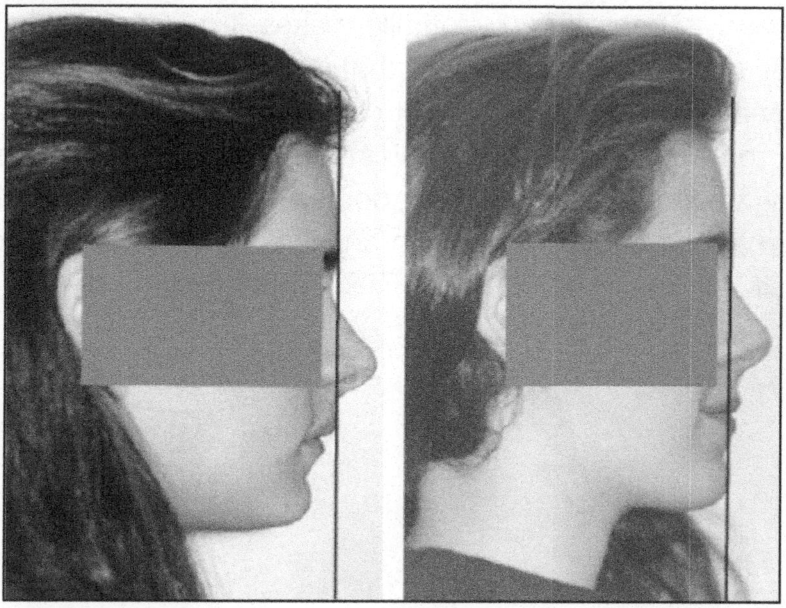

Yes, there are many appliances for jaw growth and many pages can be used to discuss this, but this book is mainly written for the public to understand the thumb suck problem and the treatment of the damages from the thumb suck habit. It isn't my place now to argue what is the best appliance and when it's to be used is, but it's that the correct diagnosis of the lower jaw is performed and that a result is truly achieved.

Sorry to say, but I see too many treatments that have failed, never attempted or diagnosed. To attempt early treatment by an orthodontic specialist or a general dentist who isn't fully trained or experienced with a severe problem mustn't be attempted or is a disservice to the patient and will hurt the profession.

I've seen patients pay as much as $4-5,000 for a so-called early treatment that basically lined up the teeth and did nothing to correct the width of the mouth that was narrow nor attempt to get the short lower jaw (retruded) to grow forward. The patient eventually makes it in my chair and I must tell them the treatment that's needed, but was never attempted. The patient in most cases and/or parent is usually in a zombie state and then states to me that they already had early treatment with another doctor yet upon examination there's a severe narrow mouth and the upper teeth stick out a half inch or more.

CHAPTER 19

Age Ten to Adult Repair of the Damage from Thumb, Finger, Toe, Blanket & Pacifier Sucking

Age Ten to Thirteen Treatment

I'll still do treatment in this age range as I will if the patient is age seven, but I have a custom consent form for the patient to sign that warns them of no refunds. I discount 30% of my age seven fee to attempt the same thing at a late age that may not work. It's the parents' choice and I basically tell them they'll pay me to try to do this with no guarantees. The hardest part is to have the cooperation of a middle school child at this age bracket.

The only step I don't like in this age group is the lower jaw growth step. If the child just turned thirteen within the past month, I'll attempt jaw growth. But, if the child is fourteen in two months, I'll decline to do it. Then, I'll treat the patient as an adult seen below in this chapter.

Age Fourteen to Adult treatment:

Mild Cases

If the open bite is 4 mm. or less there are numerous ways to attempt to close it, but it can reopen. There are new wires made from beta titanium that allow bends to be placed in these gentle wires. Elastics are used to make the front teeth come together.

It's also helpful to place an upper transpalatal arch as discussed earlier in the book. There are recent techniques with screws called temporary anchorage devices that are screwed into the bone on the inner and outer surface above the upper molars. Attached to the screws and run across the chewing surface of the upper molars are run coils to push the upper molars upward or intrude them. This decreases the wedge effect that causes the open bite and allows the front teeth to come together.

If the open bite is mild, the screws aren't usually needed and only beta titanium wires and elastics are needed as described previously.

Severe cases

Severe open bite treatment cases require braces and jaw surgery at the age of sixteen. Braces are placed one to two years (age fourteen) before the sixteenth birthday so that jaw surgery can be done at age sixteen. The bones aren't fully developed until sixteen, but you can get ready for the jaw surgery. This way, a child doesn't have braces beyond sixteen and a half. If they show up at age sixteen, they'll have braces on in their senior year of high school. No child wants this!

It usually requires the upper jaw cut into three pieces. It's not drastic because the upper jaw bone is very thin as a potato chip. Behind the upper teeth of the upper jaw are the hollow sinuses. The upper jaw isn't solid bone as the lower jaw.

A side note: I've noticed patients who require caution and need to consult with an oral surgeon highly skilled in jaw surgery before they elect jaw surgery if they have:

- **A very high palatal vault (a roof of the mouth that's a far distance from the tongue).**
- **Thin bone behind the upper four front teeth.**

The upper jaw bone in these patients can have less blood supply when they are cut. I had this one patient who required a hyperbolic oxygen tent to get oxygen to the bone structures so the bone didn't suffocate. It ended very successful and the patient didn't experience problems and was happy.

Percentages that the open bite reopens.

Caution about relapse (return to where something was) must be given to the patient and parents. Three types of open bite relapse occur:

1) I find 50% of the patients open halfway after the braces are removed.
2) 10% open all the way back to where they were.
3) 40% stay closed.

It's unpredictable who falls into what category. Patients treated with upper jaw surgery have usually a stable result and don't tend to relapse as much.

Above are nonsurgical percentages. But, things do happen in open bite cases because the tongue thrust present before braces begin can push it back open after the braces are removed. Airway or breathing problems will cause it to relapse dependent on the severity of the open bite corrected and how clear the airway is. That's why the mouth and nasal airways must be patent (cleared of obstructed items as tonsils, adenoids, mouth breathing, allergies, etc.) before treatment is started.

CHAPTER 20

Pacifier (Blinky) Habit Information & Use of the Rocky Mountain Oral Screen to Stop Thumb, Finger, Toe, Blanket & Pacifier Habits

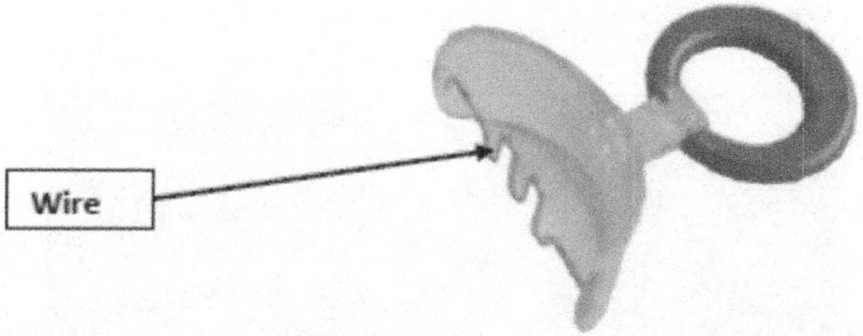

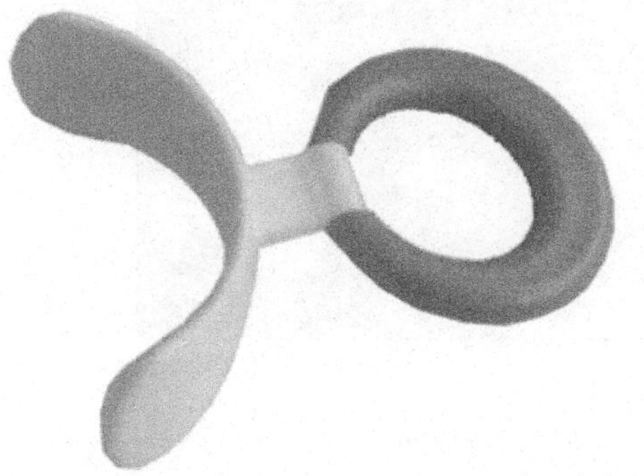

Use of the Rocky Mountain Orthodontics Oral Screen to Stop a Thumb Suck Habit

Some thumb suckers are so intense that along with my techniques in this book, I also recommend the use of the Rocky Mountain Oral Screen. These come in different designs.

I tell the thumb sucker that they'll need some additional help other than Band-Aids to help stop the urge or desire to thumb suck.

The thumb sucker patient sits in a chair across from me. The parent is present. I tell them that I have a wonderful new device or toy for them today, but we need to talk first. I talk very positive. I tell them it's the latest, coolest, newest toy or device that children use now.

Children always love the word new and they always want to have the newest device or toy especially if others have it. So, you must prepare the child and have them want this device and not tell them to use the oral screen without a proper presentation.

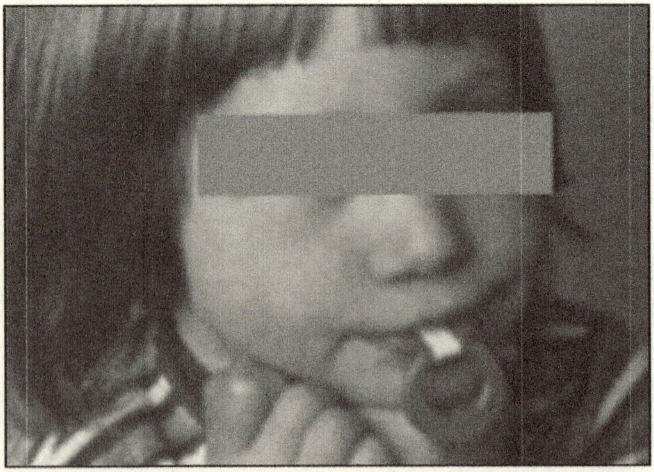

I show the above photo to the child and tell them this doesn't look bad. Again, I remind them this is no worse than a photo of them with their thumb in their mouth.

We must have 30 days straight of no thumb suck and the treatment is finished. At that time, the oral screen will stop.

I then show them the oral screen and give it to them to touch and play with. I then tell them to place it in their mouth between the lips and teeth. It's not put behind the teeth or in the tongue area. I tell them to be very careful with this device around dogs because dogs will chew it like a chew toy and destroy it within five minutes.

You'll come into a room and see it in 100 pieces. There are stories on the Internet where the family dog had surgery because they swallowed a binky and this will also apply to the oral screen. As you know, dogs will choke on many toys around the house.

The biggest pushback I get from the thumb sucker or their parent is either verbal or nonverbal communication that begs the question, "Why will I use a binky or pacifier when I need to get rid of my thumb suck habit?" I tell them, "I understand your concern, but not every thumb sucker I treat needs to do this, only if the amount done per day and the intensity of the habit necessitates extra help."

I tell the thumb sucker, "I know your thoughts right now, that I'll feel embarrassed when I have this in my mouth in the day or night." My response is, "To thumb suck is for babies up to age one. You can also use a binky or pacifier up to the age of one. It can be used as late as age two if it doesn't damage the bone structures of the mouth. So, what's the difference between when they walk around with their thumb in their mouth and a pacifier in their mouth?" The usual response from the child, parent or both is, "None."

The thumb sucker is told that they must have this on a rope or some other type of chain around the neck that won't cause them to choke if they were to fall. If they get the urge this must go in their mouth instead of the thumb. It's worn 24 hours a day. It can be removed if at school or outside the home only if no urge to suck occurs.

Use of Rocky Mountain Orthodontics Oral Screen to stop Binky or Pacifier Habits

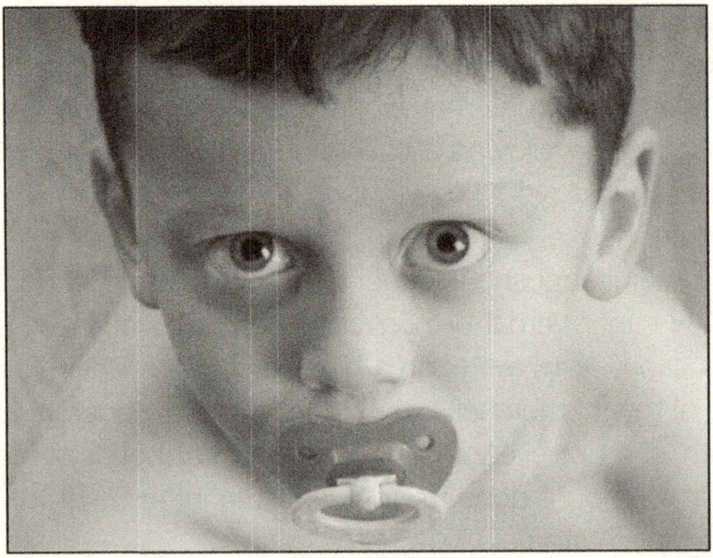

Binkies or pacifiers mustn't be used past age two. Preferably, it's best not to use it after age one. I've treated children as old as age seven that still used a pacifier. I've also treated high school student's years ago that started a fad to wear them on a chain around their neck and suck them.

The pacifier patient sits in a chair across from me. The parent is present. I tell them that I have a wonderful new device or toy for them today, but we need to talk first. I tell them that the pacifier they currently use is for babies. I asked them how old the baby is? They usually don't know the answer and will guess up to age two. I let them know that a baby is up to age one. The word baby and infant are the same. A child is older than the age of one.

I tell them that it's not only too old to use this after the age of one, but it'll cause damage to the bone and teeth. Sometimes, I'll show a photo from the Internet after I search on Google with words "Open bite photo" and then click on the word "images" to find many photos of this problem. I tell the child this will happen to your mouth if we don't get the binky out of your mouth now.

I then tell the child that I know your thoughts that you've depended on this for quite a while and its part of your life, but I have a new toy that'll help you with the urge to suck just like the binky or pacifier you currently use.

I talk very positive. I tell them it's the latest, coolest, newest toy or device that children use now. Children always love the word "new" and they always want to have the newest device or toy especially if others have it. So, you must prepare the child and have them want this device and not just take the old binky or pacifier away from them and tell them to use the oral screen without proper presentation.

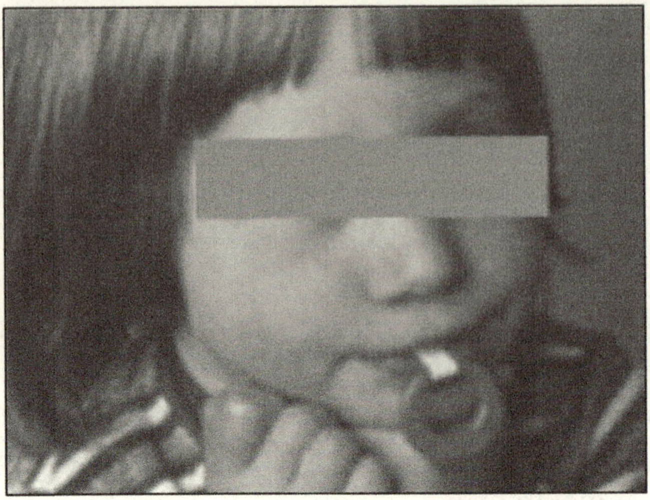

I show the above photo to the child and tell them this doesn't look bad. Again, I remind them that this is no worse than a photo of them with their thumb in their mouth. We must have 30 days straight of no binky suck and the treatment is finished. At that time, the oral screen can stop.

Use of RMO Oral Screen to stop blanket suck

Everything above applies to the blanket sucker. The presentation of the oral screen to the thumb sucker at the begin of this chapter must be done first.

It's important after the child accepts the oral screen that you let them know blanket suck harms the teeth and bone structures. Again, show them photos of an open bite on the Internet.

Tell them that you understand that the blanket has been with you for a while, but it'll disappear little by little. The best technique I've found to work is to take the blanket at a time when it isn't needed and cut a little piece of the blanket away with a pair of scissors, roughly an inch and throw it away.

What has happened in all the children I've treated with this problem is they still have the suck urge, but with use of the oral screen as a substitute technique the urge is satisfied. But, the oral screen won't hurt the bones and teeth of the mouth while at the same time their blanket disappears over a 30-day period.

Only use the next technique if you're child's upset about the blanket will disappear little by little. You bring in a second substitute while all the above is applied; allow the child to buy a stuffed animal that they can keep near and not suck on it.

How to stop use of the oral screen after thirty straight days of no habit observed

I don't tell the child in front of the parent about this. I tell the parent on the side after the techniques are done that whether you have this thought or not; you ask yourself, "How will we get the child off the oral screen since we've substituted it for the binky habit?" My first response is, "That's easy."

How do we now get the Rocky Mountain orthodontics oral screen away from the child? The technique is to alter the pacifier a little bit at a time. The oral screen design I like to use has a wire crib. By the way, there are four designs which I won't get into now.

After the child has used this for thirty days and no longer needs to suck their thumb, finger, toe, blanket or binky, the next step is to cut off the wire. The child can still suck the RMO device, but this is the first step to let the child see that this device will now start to get smaller. Eventually, alter the device until the child realizes they don't need or like it anymore.

After three days have gone by of cut the wire off, the second step is to decrease the size of the white plastic part that fits between the cheek and teeth when they suck the device. It's hard for someone at home without the tools we have in the dentist office to grind the oral screen to a smaller size.

You can find a neighbor who has some sort of grinder (called a lathe or a hand Dremel seen on Google search) to grind it down little by little, day by day. Or, go to your dentist office and have them grind it down with their grinder in the dental lab.

Also, start a substitution game with the child to begin a swap the device for some other physical item. The item depends on the age of the child. Tell the child we need you to decrease wear of this device and to help them with this we'll let them pick a new stuffed animal to have instead. It can be anything the child will play with and keep near.

If desired, the substitution can be decreased slowly. First decrease in the day and only use it fully at night and then eventually the child won't have the device at night. When it comes time to get rid of it at night, tell the child that this device was used for certain problems of the habit and those problems are for babies.

Go back through the age process again with the child to reeducate them about how old they are presently versus the age two sucker. Then, tell the child we had to use the oral screen to stop the age two problem, but the oral screen is an age zero to age one problem. Continue the discussion with the child until they decide they no longer really need this device. You may have to go back through the power processes again to get the result.

CHAPTER 21

Sample: Begin to End Treatment of a First Session Child Pacifier Sucker

Present in the room today is Beth and her mom. She's four years old and sits in a chair that faces me about 3 feet apart. Mother's been told to only answer questions directed at her and not to help the child. The mother sits behind and to the left of the child so that the child can turn and see the mother if they want to.

The back of the throat has been checked and there are no large tonsils, breathing problems or dark rings under the child's eyes. The child sleeps well and there are no home problems.

I had mom feed her protein food and no sugar or carbohydrates since it was 4 o'clock in the afternoon. She wasn't tired. You don't want to do this if the child is hungry, sleepy or had a rough day. Reschedule if things aren't perfect.

Dr. Fox: "Beth, I'm here to discuss with you about your binky (pacifier) habit. You do realize you have one, right?"

Beth: "Yes, mom has tried to get me to stop."

Dr. Fox: "I want you to look at the pictures in the front of this book and notice these people suck different things. What does this picture look like?"

Beth: "A baby."

Dr. Fox: "Great. (Continued to show 4 more photos with the same answers). Now, here are some photos (taken earlier of the sucker before the session started) that show you do the same. What does this photo look like?"

Beth: "A baby."

Dr. Fox: "Very good. I've shown you these photos of others and you to help you realize that you need to see yourself with this habit because many times I find a person with this habit only sees themselves through their eyes. They don't look at themselves from a distance while they do this habit or as if they look at themselves in a mirror while they do the habit.

Everything we're about to do and talk about over the next hour is positive. If anything I say to you sounds like it's negative or makes you feel you're a bad person, I want you to raise your right hand. I'll stop immediately and ask you what's negative.

I want you to know that from this point onward that your mother won't say anything negative to you. This includes on the way home today, tomorrow or next week like, "Look what you've done to your mouth. None of these comments help people stop the binky habit. Does this sound good to you?"

Beth: "Yes."

Dr. Fox: "The first thing we'll do is to find out when you suck the binky? Do you suck in the daytime while you're awake?"

Beth: "Yes."

Mom: "She sucks in the car."

Dr. Fox: "Thank you for your answer, but right now we'll only address the time and not places. Also, the questions are directed towards Beth so that she and I talk why you listen and we'll get your help if we need to."

Mom: "You're right, I forgot."

Dr. Fox: "Beth, let's get back to this. Do you suck your binky before you lay down to go to sleep?"

Beth: "Yes."

Dr. Fox: "Do you suck your binky before you fall asleep after you lay your head on the pillow?"

Beth: "Yes."

Dr. Fox: "Does the binky stay in your mouth after you fall asleep and through most of the night?"

Beth: "No, it falls out. I find it on the floor or in the sheets in the morning."

Dr. Fox: "Is it in your mouth when you wake up in the morning?"

Beth: "Never."

Dr. Fox: "Beth, we basically have four types of binky suckers. Someone who sucks day and night, daytime only, before bed only and nighttime only. You're a day and night binky sucker.

Now let's move on to locations where you suck your binky. We already know that you suck your binky in your sleep on the bed. Do you suck your binky when you come home from school and get on the sofa?"

Beth: "Yes."

Dr. Fox: "Do you suck your binky after you do your homework and watch television around 7:00 PM?"

Beth: "Yes."

Dr. Fox: "Do you suck your binky under the bed or in a closet with the door closed?"

Beth: "Sometimes, I'll go in the bathroom and close the door to hide from everyone and do it."

Dr. Fox: "I want to find all the places that you do this so that later in the hour we can help you not do it in those places. Do you suck your binky in the backseat of a car on a short trip to the grocery store?"

Beth: "Yes."

Dr. Fox: "Do you do it at the movie theater where it's dark and no one can see you?"

Beth: "Yes, just last week I did."

Dr. Fox: "So, it seems like you don't suck your binky anywhere where there's a chance that someone may see you do it except for others in your family, right?"

Beth: "Yes."

Dr. Fox: "So, is there anything else you want to tell me about times and locations where you suck your binky?"

Beth: "No."

Dr. Fox: "Are you okay? I haven't said anything that bothers you or made you feel bad?"

Beth: "No."

Dr. Fox: "Do you suck on a blanket before bed, while asleep or in the day?"

Beth: "No. I do sleep with a stuffed turtle that I've had for years."

Dr. Fox: "All is okay. Do you suck on pens or other objects?"

Beth: "No."

Dr. Fox: "Good. The next thing we'll do is fun. What this will do is give you the power to stop suck your binky even though you have had this power to stop before today, but didn't realize it. Let's start.

First, let's pretend that you'll go to Disney World with three of your friends this Saturday. You walk around with your three friends and have fun. Can you see or imagine this?"

Beth: "Yes."

Dr. Fox: "Will you suck your binky at Disney World with your friends?"

Beth: "No."

Dr. Fox: "Why not?"

Beth: "I don't want my friends to see me suck my binky because they'll think I'm a baby."

Dr. Fox: "Good, you made the right decision. Now, let's play a game of pretend. What if you're at Disney World with your friends 24 hours straight and you won't need to sleep. And, you won't get tired and you and your friends are on the rides. Will you suck your binky?"

Beth: "No."

Dr. Fox: "That's awesome, isn't it? So, you do have the ability to not suck your binky for 24 hours. Beth, you don't have to suck your binky, do you?"

Beth: "No."

Dr. Fox: "Beth, now let's go to something else that's fun. I want you to tell me three very important people that you have seen on TV that you'll like to meet. They can be a sports player, actor or singer."

Beth: "Carrie Underwood, Kelly Clarkson and Taylor Swift."

Dr. Fox: "Great. Now, I want you to pick one of these three that will come over tonight to sit at the dinner table beside you and they'll spend the night in your home."

Beth: "Wow, that'll have to be Taylor Swift."

Dr. Fox: "Imagine she has gotten out of her limousine and you open the front door and say hello. You have her sit beside you at the dinner table. Will you suck your binky in front of her?"

Beth: "No way."

Dr. Fox: "Why not?"

Beth: "I just won't. She'll think I'm a baby."

Dr. Fox: "She'll spend the night and sleep in your bed. Your parents will have you sleep on a cot in the same room. Will you suck your binky while Taylor's in your bedroom?"

Beth: "No."

Dr. Fox: "If she's with you 24 hours a day, you won't put your binky in your mouth, will you?"

Beth: "No."

Dr. Fox: "You then have the power to decide to carry this same thought in your mind over to every minute of the day and night and decide never to suck your binky again." (I said this while I moved my head vertically up and down to encourage a yes answer, but I don't say anything and wait for the child to say yes.)

Beth: "Yes."

Dr. Fox: "Now, let's go on to something fun, but different. Imagine you're in front of your friends at kindergarten or daycare school and you tell them about the weekend you had. While you tell them the weekend story you decide whether to put your binky in your mouth for them to see. You don't because why?"

Beth: "Because they'll call me a baby."

Dr. Fox: "That's awesome. If these friends are with you 24 hours a day you won't suck your binky, right?"

Beth: "No."

Dr. Fox: "So, you do have the power to decide to carry this same thought in your mind over to every minute of the day and night and right now to decide never to suck your binky again, right?"

Beth: "Yes."

Dr. Fox: "What's your favorite thing you like to do when you go outside and play?"

Beth: "Ride my bike with friends."

Dr. Fox: "What color is your bike?"

Beth: "Purple."

Dr. Fox: "While you ride your bike do you suck your binky?"

Beth: "No."

Dr. Fox: "Will you ride your bike 24 hours a day if you won't have to sleep?"

Beth: "Yes."

Dr. Fox: "You do have the ability to decide not to suck your binky if you think you'll ride your bike with friends 24 hours a day?"

Beth: "Yes."

Dr. Fox: "Great! We're almost finished with this step. Can you do anything about last week, last month or one year ago?"

Beth: "No."

Dr. Fox: "Can you do anything about something in five minutes from now?"

Beth: "Yes."

Dr. Fox: "Can you do anything about something next week or next month?"

Beth: "Yes."

Dr. Fox: "What's the point to all of this? There's nothing you can do about the past … only the present and future. Do you agree with this?"

Beth: "Yes. I can only do things that go on now and in the future."

Dr. Fox: "Can you do anything about suck your binky this morning, last night, yesterday, last week or last year?"

Beth: "No."

Dr. Fox: "You have the right to forgive yourself for a mistake made since everyone makes mistakes. Correct?"

Beth: "Yes."

Dr. Fox: "You have my permission to start fresh, right now and never binky suck again and pretend that it never happened since it's now only a memory. Is that okay with you?"

Beth: "Yes."

Dr. Fox: "Beth, you made the right decision. Awesome! Do you realize that you have the power to stop and start anything, control this habit and never do it again?"

Beth: "Yes, I have the ability to stop Binky suck." (This was the key answer I needed from Beth).

Dr. Fox: "Great! Let's move on to the next step that helps you in different times and places so you can help yourself not get in the situation where you feel like you need to suck the binky. We'll handle the urges that pop-up day to day and how to make those urges go away. Sound good?"

Beth: "Yes."

Dr. Fox: "We're just about half-way finished. Are you okay? You're not tired or hungry?"

Beth: "No."

Dr. Fox: "Has there been anything that I've said that sounded negative or made you feel bad?"

Beth: "No."

Dr. Fox: "We'll now go to the next step. We'll go back and forth places where you suck and don't suck your binky. Tell me where you suck your binky. Do you do it at home on the sofa when you come home from daycare or school?"

Beth: "Yes."

Dr. Fox: "Have you done it at home on a Sunday afternoon when you're tired and bored with nothing to do?"

Beth: "Yes."

Dr. Fox: "Do you suck your binky in the back seat of a car on a vacation trip or for a short trip to the grocery store?"

Beth: "Yes."

Dr. Fox: "Do you suck your binky at night when you go to bed?"

Beth: "Yes."

Dr. Fox: "Do you suck in the bed to help you fall asleep?"

Beth: "Yes."

Dr. Fox: "Now, let's go into all the places where you don't suck your binky. Do you do it in front of your friends when you're at daycare or kindergarten school?"

Beth: "No."

Dr. Fox: "Do you suck your binky when you go out to dinner with your parents?"

Beth: "No."

Dr. Fox: "How about in front of your friends at a birthday party, do you suck your binky?"

Beth: "No."

Dr. Fox: "Do you really need to suck your binky?"

Beth: "No, I don't need to suck my binky."

Dr. Fox: "You made the right decision. We're ready to go to the next step to help you not get into situations that will cause you to want to suck your binky. We'll break up your past routines where you sucked your binky.

The easiest one to start with is when you're home at 4:00 pm. I prefer that you don't watch television. Go outside and do something as long as your mom knows where you are. You can play dolls, but don't get on the sofa. Why is that?"

Beth: "If I get on the sofa, I'll get bored and suck my binky."

Dr. Fox: "Great! Your mom must give you food and drink at this time of day that won't ruin dinner.

No sugar or carbohydrates allowed. Have celery sticks, vegetables and a piece of chicken. You need to have energy and feel peppy. Many people eat lunch at noon, but they don't eat dinner until six to seven o'clock at night. That's too much time to go without food.

You told me you suck your binky before sleep. I want you very tired when you go to sleep so that you don't have to suck your binky. What time do you go to sleep?"

Beth: "7:00 PM. I get up at 6:30 AM."

Dr. Fox: "If it's okay with your mom I want you to stay up until 7:30 or 8:00 PM."

Mom: "That sounds okay."

Dr. Fox: "Mom, from 7 o'clock to 8:00 PM, I don't want her to lay on the sofa. If she watches TV, I want her to sit in a chair so that she doesn't get sleepy and the binky makes its way into the mouth. This way, she'll be tired when she goes to sleep.

Also, when you're ready to go to sleep, I want mom to pull up a chair beside your bed to give you a back massage while you turn away from her. This will help you relax and go to sleep without your binky. If she sits on your bed and gets up, you'll wake up from her leaving. Does that sound good to you Beth?"

Beth: "Yes."

Dr. Fox: "Mom, rub her shoulders and back with medium pressure and then as she's gone to sleep, barely touch her pajamas. Then, get up and tiptoe out of the room. Please don't check back on her since you don't want to wake her up. Do this for a week.

Now, let's go to the next location. The backseat of the car. For the next thirty days, we need to break up your routine. I want mom to sit in the back seat and you in the front seat as your dad drives the car. Plan B is mom sits in the backseat with you. Does this sound good, Beth?" (This all depends on child seat laws in each state. The key is to do something different.)

Beth: "Yes."

Dr. Fox: "Beth, realize that I don't want you to put yourself into situations or locations that'll make you want to suck your binky. I realize that you do know what a habit is and that it's something that you don't have to do, but for some reason you do it. Just like people who smoke cigarettes. Do you ever see people smoke cigarettes?"

Beth: "Yes."

Dr. Fox: "Do you ever see people who drink too much alcohol?"

Beth: "Yes."

Dr. Fox: "Do you ever see people who are fat and they still eat too much?"

Beth: "Yes."

Dr. Fox: "The point to all of this is that those people need to break up their routine and not put themselves in a situation that will require them to smoke, drink or eat when they don't need to. If a friend asks a person who's 100 pounds overweight to go get some ice cream with them and they're on a diet, should the friend go to the ice cream store?"

Beth: "No."

Dr. Fox: "Very good. We're now at the last step. Everything okay?"

Beth: "Yes."

Dr. Fox: "What I want to do now is help you realize key or important information about binky suck that you may or may not have thought about. Do you know what age a baby or infant is?"

Beth: "Up to age three."

Dr. Fox: "Thank you for your answer, but it's only up to age one. Do you know that you don't suck your binky past age one?"

Beth: "No."

Dr. Fox: "Do you know that binky suck is for babies up to age one?"

Beth: "No."

Dr. Fox: "Raise your right hand and show me how old you are with your fingers."

Beth: "I'm four (She holds up four fingers)."

Dr. Fox: "Good. Beth, up to what age are you able to suck your binky as a baby?"

Beth: "One."

Dr. Fox: "Use your left hand and show me with your fingers what your answer is."

Beth: "One (she holds up one finger with her left hand)."

Dr. Fox: "You have told me that you are age four and you don't suck your binky past age one and that babies are up to age one. Are you a baby and are you supposed to suck your binky at age four?"

Beth: "No, I'm not a baby and I'm not supposed to suck my binky."

Dr. Fox: "Very good answer. Now, we'll switch to something else, but very like what we just did. Will it be okay if your mother comes to daycare and sit there all day long in those tiny chairs that you sit in and do things you do?"

Beth: "No."

Dr. Fox: "Will it be okay for your dad to ride a bike that's the same size as yours along with you and your friends?"

Beth: "No."

Dr. Fox: "That will look weird because they're too old to do those things, right?"

Beth: "Yes, it'll look weird. They're too old to do that."

Dr. Fox: "Beth, is it okay for you to suck your binky if you do it past age one?"

Beth: "No."

Dr. Fox: "When someone sees you suck your binky at age four, what do you think they think?"

Beth: "They think I'm a baby or it's weird that this child sucks a binky."

Dr. Fox: "Very good answer. So, do you feel it's okay for you to suck your binky at age four anymore?"

Beth: "No."

Dr. Fox: "Will you stop suck your binky right now and never do it again?"

Beth: "Yes."

Dr. Fox: "Do you know you've hurt your teeth and they don't touch in the front?"

Beth: "Yes."

Dr. Fox: "Will you take a hammer and hit your big toe on your right foot?"

Beth: "No."

Dr. Fox: "Will you take that same hammer and hit your teeth and break them?"

Beth: "No."

Dr. Fox: "Beth, you don't use a hammer, but the binky hurts your teeth. We don't want you to hurt them anymore. Is that okay with you?"

Beth: "Yes."

Dr. Fox: "I'll help you with this. We're almost finished. I have something that'll help you not put your binky in your mouth in the day. After this, we'll go into a reward system to help you not suck your binky for thirty days. If it's not sucked for thirty days, then we know it's gone. Let's first get into the positive surprise."

Beth: "Okay."

Dr. Fox: (Turn to the Binky chapter of this book and find the photo of the child with the oral screen). "Do you like to get something new? Like a new pair of new shoes or a new bicycle?"

Beth: "Yes."

Dr. Fox: "I have the latest and newest binky that all the children now use around the world and are excited about it. It also doesn't hurt the teeth and anyone over the age of one uses it when they feel the urge. But, it helps children, your age, not need a binky after 30 days. Let me show you a picture of what it looks like.

In this picture, it still looks like your binky. It has a loop so you can add a rope to it. Keep it around your neck when you're at home. Yes, it still looks like the child in this picture is a baby, but at least it won't cause harm to the teeth because it doesn't have a nipple. Suck on it when you have the urge to suck. This is called a mouth screen (oral screen).

Every seven days the mouth screen will be reduced in size and within thirty days the only thing you'll have left is the ring.

I do have one important rule. The mouth screen isn't punishment; it's only a reminder to stop the urge to suck on any object. If you must suck, you must do it with the new mouth screen. Do you agree?"

Beth: "Yes."

Dr. Fox: "Give me your old binky so that I can give you a brand-new mouth screen. (Beth gives Dr. Fox her old binky.) Good. (I now have the oral screen in my hands, but hidden because I want Beth to be excited about the mystery of what it looks like). Beth, this comes in a little case and here it is.

Let me open the case and show you what it looks like. Again, this is the newest thing that everybody wants. Hold your hand out and touch it with both hands. Now, put it in your mouth and the plastic goes between your lips and your teeth. Don't put it behind your teeth where the tongue is. It's great, isn't it?"

Beth: "Yes, I like it."

Dr. Fox: "Give me your hand. Let's shake hands that you'll try 100% to keep the mouth screen around your neck so it's handy in case you have the urge to suck. I don't want you to leave this in the bedroom and then have an urge to suck and you're in the kitchen. It must be ready for you to use ASAP especially in the next seven days (I shook hands in agreement with Beth)."

Note #1 to reader: If you don't have the ability to order or get an oral screen, an alternative method that works is to buy a new binky and find a way to remove the nipple and smooth down the area somehow where the nipple is removed to leave the rest of the binky intact. It's very important that you buy a new binky because we don't want any reminders of the old one. In other words, a serious mistake will be to take the child's current binky, remove the nipple in front of the child or in another room and then give the old one back to the child. The child must totally disconnect from the old binky to wean the child away from the use of any oral device.

Note #2 to reader: Be prepared. You may need to practice this with a friend first since your child may cry and you won't know what to say or do. You must be a very positive mother and encourage the child. If they start to cry and get upset, tell them you understand. Don't tell them they'll get a new binky because we don't want to use that word any longer either. Tell them they'll get the newest device that all the children their age around the world now want who have this same problem and you're too old to use a binky. Tell them it'll be okay and you'll still be able to suck if you must, but we don't want you to hurt your teeth anymore.

Note #3 to reader: If the child has a severe open bite because the binky has pushed the upper and lower front teeth apart, you can get an oral screen that has a metal wavy wire (there are four designs of the oral screen). It's best to get this design so that the child will be able to bite the metal wavy wire with their back teeth to stabilize it better in the mouth. I find this very helpful. If not, you'll have to do the best you can with the design that has no wire or buy a new binky and cut off the nipple.

Dr. Fox: "The last thing is to set up a reward system because everything in life is about goals. It's easier to achieve goals if we break goals down into steps and reward each step along the way. You mustn't suck a binky with a nipple for 30 days or four weeks. At the end of each week that you didn't suck a binky with a nipple on it, a reward is decided between you and your mom. Meanwhile, you'll suck on the oral screen as it gets smaller each week.

It's best for the two of you to discuss this on the way home; your mom already has some ideas. But, I don't want you to push mom for something you want. I don't want you to change your mind what the rewards are since you need to stick to the original rewards. Then, your last week when you've reached 30 days in a row of not suck a binky with a nipple on it and your mouth screen gets thrown away, you'll get your final reward.

You'll keep a calendar on the refrigerator that has little squares. In the morning, put a check in the square for the previous day and night that you kept your oral screen near you. At night, you can put it on your night stand so not to choke on the rope.

The first week prize or award is a small item, especially if it's something you'll get anyway. If you must buy clothes for school I understand, but we mustn't buy anything for the next 30 days. No, I don't expect your mom to buy you a horse or car as your final reward. This is totally between you and her, not me.

Mom, keep her busy. I want her to do her homework, but I also want her to be creative. Play video games and on the phone, isn't creative. Go to the art store and get charcoal pencils and paper to draw things as flowers, horses or use her imagination. Singing or music lessons is another idea.

Most binky suckers are very bored, don't create enough and are very smart. We must get them to use their mind and their abilities. Find something she loves to do and is very passionate about.

Beth, we're finished. I want one last handshake that you agree 100% to keep the mouth screen on you always when you're home. I want you to call me in twenty-four hours and personally let me know how you are and how often your need to use the oral screen. Also, I want to talk to you in four to six days in person for a quick fifteen minutes and we need to set that time up now.

I'm very proud of you right now that you made the decision to use the newest oral screen. I know you'll get thirty checkmarks in a row on your calendar. Then, we'll know this habit is totally gone. I'm very proud of you. Good luck."

Note to reader: In seven days, you'll find a way to decrease the size of the oral screen by one fourth every week and by the thirteeth day, the ring will only be left. If the child asks you why you decrease the size of it, tell them that this is part of the process for you not to need this any longer. You know the binky isn't sucked after the age of one and I'm here to help you help yourself.

THE END

ABOUT THE AUTHOR

Dr. Donald Fox was born in Richmond, Virginia. It was in fourth grade, while at a picnic with Dr. William Crockett that he decided to become a doctor. Dr. Crockett, a leading instructor at the Medical College of Virginia Dental School, helped Dr. Fox focus to stay in school and become one of the most talented Orthodontists in the United States.

While in high school, Dr. Fox started to develop his diet. After he graduated from Hermitage High School, he attended the University of Richmond, Virginia and researched how to repair damaged DNA in bacteria with visible wavelengths of light. He graduated with a Bachelor of Science Degree in Chemistry.

Dr. Fox took graduate courses in histology (the study of cells), embryology (the study how cells form and how they go on to make organs and other tissues), anatomy and human physiology. It was during this time when he discovered aspi- rin and acetaminophen can cause birth defects if taken while pregnant.

Dr. Fox entered dental school, achieved numerous awards and graduated first out of a class of 115. He received The American Cancer Society Award for the highest scores on pathology examinations over a two-year period. He received the Southeastern Board of Prosthodontists Award for outstanding achievements, contributions and performance in prosthodontics (false teeth). He was recognized for his research with Dr. Robert Campbell, Oral Surgeon, of patients who experienced numbness in their lower lip and chin after jaw surgery, wisdom teeth extractions and broken jaws. For this he was awarded The American Dental Society of Anesthesiology Award.

Dr. Fox then attended the University of Tennessee and completed a residency in Orthodontics (dental braces). In his research, Dr. Fox discovered birth defects resulted from normal dosages of aspirin or acetaminophen taken during pregnancy. While there, he completed one of the lengthiest Master of Science degree theses written in the history of the university. His animal studies followed FDA birth defect protocol, so caution must be given with use of these two drugs during pregnancy. In addition to FDA protocol, Dr. Fox used radiographs to look for birth defects to set an example for future birth defect research. He also suggested that his method along with MRI, CT scans and other diagnostic tools would in the future replace the aged techniques used by the FDA.

Dr. Fox was also awarded the Chairman's Research Award in Orthodontics and the Woodrow Powell Research Award for recognition of an original research investigation, which had produced unique and significant knowledge for the specialty of Orthodontics.

The American Association of Orthodontists awarded him the American Association of Orthodontists Harry Sicher Award for the most meritorious first research in the United States and Canada. His research was then presented at the annual meeting of The American Association of Orthodontists in New Orleans and at the annual meeting of The Growth Symposium at the University of Michigan.

Dr. Fox has a Master of Science degree in Orthodontics and Dentofacial Orthopedics. This encompasses dental braces that straighten the teeth and jaws and the ability to change the shape, length and width of the jaws of the face. This is done as early as age seven with non-surgical methods or in the teenage and adult years with non-surgical and surgical methods.

Dr. Fox went into private practice where he has written more than 200 articles in dentistry that help administrative staff, assistants and patients plus manuals for different job positions in Dentistry. He has produced more than 120 educational videos.

He has developed techniques that decrease the urge to gag or choke when dental impressions of the mouth are performed. Also, Dr. Fox has tested the glue used to stick braces onto the teeth. He recently completed research on how to tolerate extreme heat with the use of salt and potassium. He has identified four new stages of heat exhaustion. This will help people who work or play sports in extreme heat to recognize early stages of heat exhaustion much sooner than presented previously. Dr. Fox also developed methods to repair the early stages. His primary focus is now on racecar drivers, their pit crews and football players.

In his spare time, Dr. Fox goes to NASCAR races, football games and hockey games. He collects sports memorabilia and loves to travel.

He has contributed large donations to the Clearwater Aquarium in Clearwater, Florida, to help with research and the salvage of stranded and hurt marine wildlife, particularly sea turtles, dolphins and otters.

Dr. Fox worked personally with NASCAR to help raise over $500,000 to help pay for neonatal beds for the Homestead Hospital pediatric department. These beds cost $25,000 each and there were none at the hospital before this event causing parents to travel each day to hospitals in Miami after work to see their newborn children. These children needed their parents closer to them with their medical problems that required them to be in these neonatal beds.

Dr. Fox will continue to help others achieve their best. He knows that if he does this, it will make him a better person and doctor, but more importantly, it will better humanity.

LITERATURE REVIEW

Thumb-Sucking, Nail-Biting, and Atopic Sensitization, Asthma, and Hay Fever. Lynch SJ, Sears MR, Hancox RJ.

Pediatrics. 2016 Aug;138(2).

Hypnotic intervention in a 7-year-old thumbsucker: a case study. Grayson DN. Am J Clin Hypn. 2012 Jan;54(3):195-201.

Soothing methods used to calm a baby in an Arab country. Abdulrazzaq YM, Al Kendi A, Nagelkerke N.

Acta Paediatr. 2009 Feb;98(2):392-6.

[Psychology and dentofacial orthopedics. Apropos of various results]. Mairesse AM, Coutand A, Bouvet JM.

Rev Stomatol Chir Maxillofac. 1977;78(4):259-68. French.

Comparison of Sucking Pattern in Premature Infants With Different Feeding Methods. Rahman MA, Subramanian S, Kandraju H, Murki S. Indian Pediatr. 2015 Nov;52(11):961-3.

[Finger or thumb sucking. New interpretations and therapeutic implications]. Ferrante A, Ferrante A. Minerva Pediatr. 2015 Aug;67(4):285-97. Italian.

The promotion of exclusive breastfeeding in infants with complete cleft lip and palate during the first 6 months after childbirth at Srinagarind Hospital, Khon Kaen Province, Thailand. Pathumwiwatana P, Tongsukho S, Naratippakorn T, Pradubwong S, Chusilp K. J Med Assoc Thai. 2010 Oct;93 Suppl 4:S71-7.

RURS' elbow guard: an innovative treatment of the thumb-sucking habit in a child with Hurler's syndrome.

Shetty RM, Dixit U, Hegde R, Shivprakash PK. J Indian Soc Pedod Prev Dent. 2010 Jul-Sep;28(3):212-8.

[Prevalence and factors associated with non-nutritive sucking behavior. Cross sectional study among 5- to 6-year-old Senegalese children]. Ngom PI, Diagne F, Samba Diouf J, Ndiaye A, Hennequin M. Orthod Fr. 2008 Jun;79(2):99-106.

Prevalence of primitive reflexes and the relationship with cognitive change in healthy adults: a report from the Maastricht Aging Study. van Boxtel MP, Bosma H, Jolles J, Vreeling FW. J Neurol. 2006 Jul;253(7):935-41. Epub 2006 Mar 6.

Finger sucking and onycholysis in an infant. Wu E, Viegas SF. J Hand Surg Am. 2005 May;30(3):620-2.

Implementing the Baby Friendly Hospital Initiative: the role of finger feeding. Oddy WH, Glenn K.

Breastfeed Rev. 2003 Mar;11(1):5-10.

The effect of oral-gustatory, tactile-bucal, and tactile-manual stimulation on the behavior of the hands in newborns.

Tudella E, Oishi J, Puglia Bergamasco NH. Dev Psychobiol. 2000 Sep;37(2):82-9.

Therapeutic teat use for babies who breastfeed poorly. Noble R, Bovey A. Breastfeed Rev. 1997;5(2):37-42.

Damage to the primary dentition resulting from thumb and finger (digit) sucking. Fukuta O, Braham RL, Yokoi K, Kurosu K. ASDC J Dent Child. 1996 Nov-Dec;63(6):403-7.

Program to eliminate thumb (or finger) sucking. Pierce RB. Int J Orofacial Myology. 1994 Nov;20:52-3.

[Utilization of pacifiers: distribution, causes and sequelae]. Peters N. Schweiz Rundsch Med Prax. 1993 Aug 17;82(33):885-7. German.

Sucking habits and occlusion in 3-year-old children. Ravn JJ. Scand J Dent Res. 1976 Jul;84(4):204-9.

Oral sucking habits among children with Down syndrome and cerebral palsy. Carneiro NCR, Monteiro LR, Pordeus IA, Borges-Oliveira AC. Spec Care Dentist. 2017 Jul;37(4):176-180.

Risk Factors associated with Early Childhood Caries. Sun HB, Zhang W, Zhou XB. Chin J Dent Res. 2017;20(2):97-104.

Association between harmful oral habits and the structures and functions of the stomatognathic system: perception of parents/guardians. Pereira TS, Oliveira F, Cardoso MCAF. Codas. 2017 May 15;29(3):e20150301.

Infant and Child Oral Health Risk Status Correlated to Behavioral Habits of Parents or Caregivers: A Survey in Central Italy. Vozza I, Capasso F, Marrese E, Polimeni A, Ottolenghi L. J Int Soc Prev Community Dent. 2017 Mar-Apr;7(2):95-99.

"Media Addiction" in a 10-Year-Old Boy. Brown S, Scharf MA, Bustos C, Chavira D, Stein MT. J Dev Behav Pediatr. 2017 Feb/Mar;38 Suppl 1:S69-S72.

Non-nutritive sucking habits and their effects on the occlusion in the deciduous dentition in children. Lopes Freire GM, Espasa Suarez de Deza JE, Rodrigues da Silva IC, Butini Oliveira L, Ustrell Torrent JM, Boj Quesada JR.

Eur J Paediatr Dent. 2016 Dec;17(4):301-306.

[Effects of breast-feeding duration, bottle-feeding duration and oral habits on the occlusal characteristics of primary dentition]. Chen XX, Xia B, Ge LH, Yuan JW. Beijing Da Xue Xue Bao. 2016 Dec 18;48(6):1060-1066. Chinese.

Are distinctive risk indicators associated with different stages of caries in children? A cross-sectional study.

Cagetti MG, Congiu G, Cocco F, Meloni G, Sale S, Campus G. BMC Public Health. 2016 Dec 1;16(1):1213.

Evaluation of a preventive educational program for malocclusions: 7-year study. Scarpelli BB, Berger SB, Punhagui MF, Oliveira CA, Ferelle A, Oltramari-Navarro PV. Braz Oral Res. 2016 Nov 28;30(1):e119.

Factors associated with malocclusion in youth in a municipality of Northeastern Brazil. Teixeira AK, Antunes JL, Noro LR. Rev Bras Epidemiol. 2016 Jul-Sep;19(3):621-631.

Children using Day Nurseries' Facilities can be Associated with more Risk to Nonnutritive Sucking Habits.

Alves FB, Wambier DS, Alvarez JH, da Rocha JC, Kummer TR, de Castro VC, Cabral H, Kozlowski VA Jr.

J Contemp Dent Pract. 2016 Sep 1;17(9):721-727.

Establishing the association between nonnutritive sucking behavior and malocclusions: A systematic review and meta-analysis. Doğramacı EJ, Rossi-Fedele G. J Am Dent Assoc. 2016 Dec;147(12):926-934.e6. doi: 10.1016/j.adaj.2016.08.018. Epub 2016 Sep 28. Review.

Familial and dietary risk factors in Early Childhood Caries. Paglia L, Scaglioni S, Torchia V, De Cosmi V, Moretti M, Marzo G, Giuca MR. Eur J Paediatr Dent. 2016 Jun;17(2):93-9.

Interference of conventional and orthodontic nipples in system stomatognathmedia addictionic: systematic review. Corrêa Cde C, Bueno Mda R, Lauris JR, Berretin-Felix G. Codas. 2016 Apr;28(2):182-9. doi: 10.1590/2317-1782/ 20162015024. Review. English, Portuguese.

Early risk factors for posterior crossbite and anterior open bite in the primary dentition. Germa A, Clément C, Weissenbach M, Heude B, Forhan A, Martin-Marchand L, Bonet M, Vital S, Kaminski M, Nabet C. Angle Orthod. 2016 Sep;86(5):832-8.

Anterior open-bite and sucking habits in Italian preschool children. Silvestrini-Biavati A, Salamone S, Silvestrini-Biavati F, Agostino P, Ugolini A. Eur J Paediatr Dent. 2016 Mar;17(1):43-6.

Prevalence and Predictors of Early Childhood Caries in 3- to 6-year-old South Indian Children--A Cross-sectional Descriptive Study. Gopal S, Chandrappa V, Kadidal U, Rayala C, Vegesna M. Oral Health Prev Dent. 2016;14(3):267-73.

Effects of conventional and orthodontic pacifiers on the dental occlusion of children aged 24-36 months old.

Lima AA, Alves CM, Ribeiro CC, Pereira AL, da Silva AA, Silva LF, Thomaz EB. Int J Paediatr Dent. 2017 Mar;27(2):108-119.

Exploring the association between feeding habits, non-nutritive sucking habits, and malocclusions in the deciduous dentition. Lopes-Freire GM, Cárdenas AB, Suarez de Deza JE, Ustrell-Torrent JM, Oliveira LB, Boj Quesada JR Jr.

Prog Orthod. 2015;16:43.

Pacifier Use, Finger Sucking, and Infant Sleep. Butler R, Moore M, Mindell JA. Behav Sleep Med. 2016 Nov-Dec;14(6):615-23.

Microbial contamination and disinfection methods of pacifiers. Nelson-Filho P, Louvain MC, Macari S, Lucisano MP, Silva RA, Queiroz AM, Gaton-Hernández P, Silva LA. J Appl Oral Sci. 2015 Oct;23(5):523-8.

Frühkindliche kieferorthopädische Therapie mittels Schnuller? Filippi C, Filippi A, Verna C. Swiss Dent J. 2015;125(9):959-70. French, German.

Occlusal characteristics in 3-year-old children--results of a birth cohort study. Wagner Y, Heinrich-Weltzien R.

BMC Oral Health. 2015 Aug 7;15:94.

Social and Behavioral Determinants for Early Childhood Caries among Preschool Children in India.

Jain M, Namdev R, Bodh M, Dutta S, Singhal P, Kumar A. J Dent Res Dent Clin Dent Prospects. 2015 Spring;9(2):115-20. doi: 10.15171/joddd.2014.023. Epub 2015 Jun 10.

Comparison between Clinical Aspects and Salivary Microbial Profile of Children with and without Early Childhood Caries: A Preliminary

Study. Neves AB, Lobo LA, Pinto KC, Pires ES, Requejo M, Maia LC, Antonio AG.

J Clin Pediatr Dent. 2015 Spring;39(3):209-14.

Lethal Lullabies: A History of Opium Use in Infants. Obladen M. J Hum Lact. 2016 Feb;32(1):75-85.

Exclusive Breastfeeding and Risk of Dental Malocclusion. Peres KG, Cascaes AM, Peres MA, Demarco FF, Santos IS, Matijasevich A, Barros AJ. Pediatrics. 2015 Jul;136(1):e60-7.

Prevalence of Non-Nutritive Sucking Habits and Potential Influencing Factors among Children in Urban Communities in Nigeria. Orimadegun AE, Obokon GO. Front Pediatr. 2015 Apr 20;3:30.

Association of breastfeeding and three-dimensional dental arch relationships in primary dentition.

Sum FH, Zhang L, Ling HT, Yeung CP, Li KY, Wong HM, Yang Y. BMC Oral Health. 2015 Mar 10;15:30.

Interventions for the cessation of non-nutritive sucking habits in children. Borrie FR, Bearn DR, Innes NP, Iheozor-Ejiofor Z. Cochrane Database Syst Rev. 2015 Mar 31;(3):CD008694.

Pacifier-sucking habit duration and frequency on occlusal and myofunctional alterations in preschool children.

Nihi VS, Maciel SM, Jarrus ME, Nihi FM, Salles CL, Pascotto RC, Fujimaki M. Braz Oral Res. 2015;29:1-7.

Prolonged pacifier use during infancy and smoking initiation in adolescence: evidence from a historical cohort study. Ferreira HR, Rosa EF, Antunes JL, Duarte DA, Imparato JC, Pannuti CM, Mendes FM. Eur Addict Res. 2015;21(1):33-8.

Prevalence and associated factors for the development of anterior open bite and posterior crossbite in the primary dentition. de Sousa RV, Ribeiro GL, Firmino RT, Martins CC, Granville-Garcia AF, Paiva SM. Braz Dent J. 2014;25(4):336-42.

Longitudinal study of habits leading to malocclusion development in childhood. Moimaz SA, Garbin AJ, Lima AM, Lolli LF, Saliba O, Garbin CA. BMC Oral Health. 2014 Aug 4;14:96

Factors associated with prolonged non-nutritive sucking habits in two cohorts of Brazilian children. Maia-Nader M, Silva de Araujo Figueiredo C, Pinheiro de Figueiredo F, Moura da Silva AA, Thomaz EB, Saraiva MC, Barbieri MA, Bettiol H. BMC Public Health. 2014 Jul 22;14:743.

Breastfeeding and sucking habits in children enrolled in a mother-child health program. Lopes TS, Moura Lde F, Lima MC. BMC Res Notes. 2014 Jun 14;7:362.

The risks of not breastfeeding: new associations. Lawrence RA. Breastfeed Med. 2014 Jun;9(5):237-8.

[Prevalence of non-nutritive sucking habits in preschoolers and parents' perception of its relationship with malocclusions]. Garbin CA, Garbin AJ, Martins RJ, Souza NP, Moimaz SA. Cien Saude Colet. 2014 Feb;19(2):553-8. Portuguese.

Breastfeeding and parafunctional oral habits in children with and without attention-deficit/hyperactivity disorder.

Sabuncuoglu O, Orengul C, Bikmazer A, Kaynar SY. Breastfeed Med. 2014 Jun;9(5):244-50

Risk factors in the mother-child relationship that predispose to the development of early childhood caries.

Moimaz SA, Garbin AJ, Lima AM, Lolli LF, Saliba O, Garbin CA. Eur Arch Paediatr Dent. 2014 Aug;15(4):245-50.

Cessation age of breast-feeding and pacifier use is associated with persistent finger-sucking. Fukumoto E, Fukumoto S, Kawasaki K, Furugen R, Kitamura M, Kawashita Y, Hayashida H, Fukuda H, Iijima Y, Saito T. Pediatr Dent. 2013;35(7):506-9.

Association between feeding methods and sucking habits: a cross-sectional study of infants in their first 18 months of life. Yonezu T, Arano-Kojima T, Kumazawa K, Shintani S. Bull Tokyo Dent Coll. 2013;54(4):215-21.

Baby-friendly hospital initiative: evaluation of the ten steps to successful breastfeeding. Lopes Sda S, Laignier MR, Primo CC, Leite FM. Rev Paul Pediatr. 2013 Dec;31(4):488-93.

Website Babies Portal: development and evaluation of the contents regarding orofacial functions. Corrêa Cde C, Pauleto AR, Ferrari DV, Berretin-Felix G. J Appl Oral Sci. 2013 Nov-Dec;21(6):581-9.

Oral habits in a population of Albanian growing subjects. Laganà G, Fabi F, Abazi Y, Beshiri Nastasi E, Vinjolli F, Cozza P. Eur J Paediatr Dent. 2013 Dec;14(4):309-13.

Oral habits as risk factors for anterior open bite in the deciduous and mixed dentition - cross-sectional study.

Urzal V, Braga AC, Ferreira AP. Eur J Paediatr Dent. 2013 Dec;14(4):299-302.

Dental caries and oral health-related factors in a sample of Greek preschool children. Boka V, Trikaliotis A, Kotsanos N, Karagiannis V. Eur Arch Paediatr Dent. 2013 Dec;14(6):363-8.

Analysis models for variables associated with breastfeeding duration. dos S Neto ET, Zandonade E, Emmerich AO.

Rev Paul Pediatr. 2013 Sep;31(3):306-14.

Early childhood caries and associated determinants: a cross-sectional study on Italian preschool children.

Congiu G, Campus G, Sale S, Spano G, Cagetti MG, Lugliè PF. J Public Health Dent. 2014 Spring;74(2):147-52.

Interceptive orthodontics--current evidence-based best practice. Borrie F, Bearn D. Dent Update. 2013 Jul-Aug;40(6):442-4, 446-8, 450.

Association of breastfeeding, pacifier use, breathing pattern and malocclusions in preschoolers. Bueno SB, Bittar TO, Vazquez Fde L, Meneghim MC, Pereira AC. Dental Press J Orthod. 2013 Feb 15;18(1):30.e1-6.

Maternal education, dental visits and age of pacifier withdrawal: pediatric dentist role in malocclusion prevention.

Pérez-Suárez V, Carrillo-Diaz M, Crego A, Romero M. J Clin Pediatr Dent. 2013 Spring;37(3):315-9.

Influence of breastfeeding on children's oral skills. Silveira LM, Prade LS, Ruedell AM, Haeffner LS, Weinmann AR. Rev Saude Publica. 2013 Feb;47(1):37-43. English, Portuguese.

Prevalence of oral habits in children with cleft lip and palate. Barsi PC, Ribeiro da Silva T, Costa B, da Silva Dalben G. Plast Surg Int. 2013;2013:247908.

Prevalence and factors associated with anterior open bite in 2 to 5-year-old children in Benin city, Nigeria.

Ize-Iyamu IN, Isiekwe MC. Afr Health Sci. 2012 Dec;12(4):446-51.

The prevalence of anterior open bite in Portuguese children during deciduous and mixed dentition--correlations for a prevention strategy. Urzal V, Braga AC, Ferreira AP. Int Orthod. 2013 Mar;11(1):93-103.

Understanding the relationships between breastfeeding, malocclusion, ADHD, sleep-disordered breathing and traumatic dental injuries. Sabuncuoglu O. Med Hypotheses. 2013 Mar;80(3):315-20.

Prevalence of malocclusion and related oral habits in 5- to 6-year-old children. dos Santos RR, Nayme JG, Garbin AJ, Saliba N, Garbin CA, Moimaz SA. Oral Health Prev Dent. 2012;10(4):311-8.

Malocclusion and deleterious oral habits among adolescents in a developing area in northeastern Brazil.

Thomaz EB, Cangussu MC, Assis AM. Braz Oral Res. 2013 Jan-Feb;27(1):62-9. Epub 2012 Dec 4.

Is breastfeeding duration influenced by maternal attitude and knowledge? A longitudinal study during the first year of life. Bertino E, Varalda A, Magnetti F, Di Nicola P, Cester E, Occhi L, Perathoner C, Soldi A, Prandi G. J Matern Fetal Neonatal Med. 2012 Oct;25 Suppl 3:32-6.

Duration of breastfeeding and distoclusion in the deciduous dentition. Caramez da Silva F, Justo Giugliani ER, Capsi Pires S. Breastfeed Med. 2012 Dec;7(6):464-8.

[Pacifier sucking habit and associated dental changes. Importance of early diagnosis]. Franco Varas V, Gorritxo Gil B. An Pediatr (Barc). 2012 Dec;77(6):374-80. doi: 10.1016/j.anpedi.2012.02.020. Epub 2012 May 18. Spanish.

A longitudinal study of the association between breast-feeding and harmful oral habits. Moimaz SA, Saliba O, Lolli LF, Garbin CA, Garbin AJ, Saliba NA. Pediatr Dent. 2012 Mar-Apr;34(2):117-21.

The oral health environment and the equal environment assumption (EEA) among 1-8-year-old twins. Holst D, Aas JA. Eur J Paediatr Dent. 2012 Mar;13(1):41-5.

Maternal breastfeeding, parafunctional oral habits and malocclusion in adolescents: a multivariate analysis. Thomaz EB, Cangussu MC, Assis AM. Int J Pediatr Otorhinolaryngol. 2012 Apr;76(4):500-6

Feeding and oral hygiene habits of children attending daycare centres in Bangalore and their caretaker's oral health knowledge, attitude and practices. Vinay S, Naveen N, Naganandini N. Indian J Dent Res. 2011 Jul-Aug;22(4):561-6.

Malocclusions and non-nutritive sucking habits: a preliminary study. Luzzi V, Guaragna M, Ierardo G, Saccucci M, Consoli G, Vestri AR, Polimeni A. Prog Orthod. 2011 Nov;12(2):114-8.

Bottle feeding, increased overjet and Class 2 primary canine relationship: is there any association? Jabbar NS, Bueno AB, Silva PE, Scavone-Junior H, Inês Ferreira R. Braz Oral Res. 2011 Jul-Aug;25(4):331-7.

Traumatic dental injuries and their association with malocclusion in the primary dentition of Irish children.

Norton E, O'Connell AC. Dent Traumatol. 2012 Feb;28(1):81-6.

[The relation between maternal breast feeding and non-nutritive sucking habits]. Moimaz SA, Rocha NB, Garbin AJ, Saliba O. Cien Saude Colet. 2011 May;16(5):2477-84. Portuguese.

Recreational strategies for the elimination of pacifier and finger sucking habits. Muzulan CF, Gonçalves MI.

J Soc Bras Fonoaudiol. 2011 Mar;23(1):66-70. English, Portuguese.

Breastfeeding and non-nutritive sucking patterns related to the prevalence of anterior open bite in primary dentition.

Romero CC, Scavone-Junior H, Garib DG, Cotrim-Ferreira FA, Ferreira RI. J Appl Oral Sci. 2011 Apr;19(2):161-8.

Non-nutritive sucking habits, anterior open bite and associated factors in Brazilian children aged 30-59 months.

Vasconcelos FM, Massoni AC, Heimer MV, Ferreira AM, Katz CR, Rosenblatt A. Braz Dent J. 2011;22(2):140-5.

Factors associated to bruxism in children from 4-6 years. Simões-Zenari M, Bitar ML. Pro Fono. 2010 Oct-Dec;22(4):465-72. English, Portuguese.

Association between sociodemographic factors and nutritive and non-nutritive sucking habits among Iranian girls.

Jahanbin A, Mokhber N, Jabbarimani A. East Mediterr Health J. 2010 Nov;16(11):1143-7.

Influence of the mode of nutritive and non-nutritive sucking on the dimensions of primary dental arches. Diouf JS, Ngom PI, Badiane A, Cisse B, Ndoye C, Diop-Ba K, Diagne F. Int Orthod. 2010 Dec;8(4):372-85

Confirmational study: a positive-based thumb and finger sucking elimination program. Green SE.

Int J Orofacial Myology. 2010 Nov; 36:44-59.

[Infant botulism in France, 1991-2009]. King LA, Popoff MR, Mazuet C, Espié E, Vaillant V, de Valk H.

Arch Pediatr. 2010 Sep;17(9):1288-92. doi: 10.1016/j.arcped.2010.06.010. Epub 2010 Aug 17. French.

Effects of feeding on non-nutritive sucking habits and implications on occlusion in mixed dentition. Montaldo L, Montaldo P, Cuccaro P, Caramico N, Minervini G. Int J Paediatr Dent. 2011 Jan;21(1):68-73.

Posterior crossbite in the deciduous dentition period, its relation with sucking habits, irregular orofacial functions, and otolaryngological findings. Melink S, Vagner MV, Hocevar-Boltezar I, Ovsenik M. Am J Orthod Dentofacial Orthop. 2010 Jul;138(1):32-40.

Maximal bite force, facial morphology and sucking habits in young children with functional posterior crossbite.

Castelo PM, Gavião MB, Pereira LJ, Bonjardim LR. J Appl Oral Sci. 2010 Mar-Apr;18(2):143-8.

Feeding and nonnutritive sucking habits and prevalence of open bite and crossbite in children/adolescents with Down syndrome. Oliveira AC, Pordeus IA, Torres CS, Martins MT, Paiva SM. Angle Orthod. 2010 Jul;80(4):748-53

[The influence of feeding methods in the development of nonnutritive sucking habits in childhood]. de Albuquerque SS, Duarte RC, Cavalcanti AL, Beltrão Ede M. Cien Saude Colet. 2010 Mar;15(2):371-8.

[Pacifier, Nuggi, thumbsucking: when should a child stop?]. Meyer J, van Waes H, Steffen R.

Kinderkrankenschwester. 2010 Mar;29(3):91-3. German

Attitudes of Saudi mothers towards prolonged non-nutritive sucking habits in children. Al-Hussyeen AJ.

Saudi Dent J. 2010 Apr;22(2):77-82.

Effect of breast- and bottle-feeding duration on the age of pacifier use persistence. Telles FB, Ferreira RI, Magalhães Ldo N, Scavone-Junior H. Braz Oral Res. 2009 Oct-Dec;23(4):432-8.

Pacifier habit: history and multidisciplinary view. Castilho SD, Rocha MA. J Pediatr (Rio J). 2009 Nov-Dec;85(6):480-9.

Relationship between breast- and bottle-feeding and non-nutritive sucking habits. de Holanda AL, dos Santos SA, Fernandes de Sena M, Ferreira MA. Oral Health Prev Dent. 2009;7(4):331-7.

Pacifier-sucking and breast-feeding: a comparison between the 1960 s and the 1990 s. Lindsten R, Larsson E.

J Dent Child (Chic). 2009 Sep-Dec;76(3):199-203.

Do sucking habits in preschool children influence the position of the primary incisors? Abrahão GM, Fernandes DJ, Miguel JA, Quintão C, de Oliveira BH. World J Orthod. 2009 Fall;10(3):229-32.

Anterior open bite: a case-control study. Heimer MV, Katz CR, Rosenblatt A. Int J Paediatr Dent. 2010 Jan;20(1):59-64

The relationship of bottle feeding and other sucking behaviors with speech disorder in Patagonian preschoolers.

Barbosa C, Vasquez S, Parada MA, Gonzalez JC, Jackson C, Yanez ND, Gelaye B, Fitzpatrick AL.

BMC Pediatr. 2009 Oct 21;9:66

Nonnutritive sucking habits among preschool-aged children. Santos SA, Holanda AL, Sena MF, Gondim LA, Ferreira MA. J Pediatr (Rio J). 2009 Sep-Oct;85(5):408-14

Incorrect orofacial functions until 5 years of age and their association with posterior crossbite. Ovsenik M. Am J Orthod Dentofacial Orthop. 2009 Sep;136(3):375-81

Non-nutritive sucking habits in sleeping infants. Hanzer M, Zotter H, Sauseng W, Pichler G, Muller W, Kerbl R.

Neonatology. 2010;97(1):61-6

Self-inflicted gingival injury due to habitual fingernail scratching: a case report with a 1-year follow up. Dilsiz A, Aydin T. Eur J Dent. 2009 Apr;3(2):150-4.

Prevalence of a posterior crossbite and sucking habits in Brazilian children aged 18-59 months. Macena MC, Katz CR, Rosenblatt A. Eur J Orthod. 2009 Aug;31(4):357-61.

Relationship between malocclusion and behavioral, demographic and socioeconomic variables: a cross-sectional study of 5-year-olds. Hebling SR, Cortellazzi KL, Tagliaferro EP, Hebling E, Ambrosano GM, Meneghim Mde C, Pereira AC. J Clin Pediatr Dent. 2008 Fall;33(1):75-9.

Oral conditions in very low and extremely low birth weight children. Ferrini FR, Marba ST, Gavião MB.

J Dent Child (Chic). 2008 Sep-Dec;75(3):235-42.

Trichotillomania in early childhood--a report of two cases with a peculiar habit. Madsen JT, Bygum A.

Pediatr Dermatol. 2008 Sep-Oct;25(5):575-6.

Association between breast-feeding practices and sucking habits: a cross-sectional study of children in their first year of life. Moimaz SA, Zina LG, Saliba NA, Saliba O. J Indian Soc Pedod Prev Dent. 2008 Sep;26(3):102-6.

Association between breastfeeding duration and non-nutritive sucking habits. Scavone-Jr H, Guimarães-Jr CH, Ferreira RI, Nahás AC, Vellini-Ferreira F. Community Dent Health. 2008 Sep;25(3):161-5.

Caries prevalence in 2-year-old children in the city of Zurich. Menghini G, Steiner M, Thomet E, Roos M, Imfeld T.

Community Dent Health. 2008 Sep;25(3):154-60.

Longitudinal study on influence of prolonged non-nutritive sucking habits on dental caries in Japanese children from 1.5 to 3 years of age. Yonezu T, Yakushiji M. Bull Tokyo Dent Coll. 2008 May;49(2):59-63.

Non-nutritive sucking habits, dental malocclusions, and facial morphology in Brazilian children: a longitudinal study. Heimer MV, Tornisiello Katz CR, Rosenblatt A. Eur J Orthod. 2008 Dec;30(6):580-5

Thumb and finger sucking. Davidson L. Pediatr Rev. 2008 Jun;29(6):207-8

Allergic rhinitis, feeding and oral habits, toothbrushing and socioeconomic status. Effects on development of dental caries in primary dentition. Vázquez-Nava F, Vázquez RE, Saldivar GA, Beltrán GF, Almeida AV, Vázquez RC.

Caries Res. 2008;42(2):141-7.

Sucking habits in childhood and the effects on the primary dentition: findings of the Avon Longitudinal Study of Pregnancy and Childhood. Duncan K, McNamara C, Ireland AJ, Sandy JR. Int J Paediatr Dent. 2008 May;18(3):178-88. doi: 10.1111/j.1365-263X.2007.00905.x. Epub 2008 Mar 6.

Influence of nonnutritive sucking habits, breathing pattern and adenoid size on the development of malocclusion.

Góis EG, Ribeiro-Júnior HC, Vale MP, Paiva SM, Serra-Negra JM, Ramos-Jorge ML, Pordeus IA. Angle Orthod. 2008 Jul;78(4):647-54.

Follow-up study of functional and morphological malocclusion trait changes from 3 to 12 years of age. Ovsenik M, Farcnik FM, Korpar M, Verdenik I. Eur J Orthod. 2007 Oct;29(5):523-9.

Occlusal and orofacial myofunctional evaluation in children with anterior open bite before and after removal of pacifier sucking habit. Verrastro AP, Stefani FM, Rodrigues CR, Wanderley MT.

Int J Orthod Milwaukee. 2007 Fall;18(3):19-25.

The advantages and disadvantages of pacifier use. Cinar DN. Contemp Nurse. 2004 Jul-Aug;17(1-2):109-12. Review.

Transverse features of subjects with sucking habits and facial hyperdivergency in the mixed dentition.

Cozza P, Baccetti T, Franchi L, Mucedero M, Polimeni A. Am J Orthod Dentofacial Orthop. 2007 Aug;132(2):226-9.

For the dental patient. Thumb sucking and pacifier use. [No authors listed] J Am Dent Assoc. 2007 Aug;138(8):1176.

Occlusal and orofacial myofunctional evaluation in children with primary dentition, anterior open bite and pacifier sucking habit.

Verrastro AP, Stefani FM, Rodrigues CR, Wanderley MT. Int J Orofacial Myology. 2006 Nov;32:7-21.

Prevalence of posterior crossbite among pacifier users: a study in the deciduous dentition. Scavone H Jr, Ferreira RI, Mendes TE, Ferreira FV. Braz Oral Res. 2007 Apr-Jun;21(2):153-8.

Effects of breastfeeding and sucking habits on malocclusion in a birth cohort study. Peres KG, Barros AJ, Peres MA, Victora CG. Rev Saude Publica. 2007 Jun;41(3):343-50.

Finger habits: their effects and their treatments--part 2. Bishara SE, Larsson E. Dent Assist. 2007 Mar-Apr;76(2):16-8, 20, 22 passim.

Frequency of parafunctional oral habits in patients with cerebral palsy. Ortega AO, Guimarães AS, Ciamponi AL, Marie SK. J Oral Rehabil. 2007 May;34(5):323-8.

Effects of pacifiers on early oral development. Poyak J. Int J Orthod Milwaukee. 2006 Winter;17(4):13-6.

Social and biological early life influences on the prevalence of open bite in Brazilian 6-year-olds. Peres KG, De Oliveira Latorre Mdo R, Sheiham A, Peres MA, Victora CG, Barros FC. Int J Paediatr Dent. 2007 Jan;17(1):41-9.

Association of maternal-child characteristics as a factor in early childhood caries and salivary bacterial counts.

Ersin NK, Eronat N, Cogulu D, Uzel A, Aksit S. J Dent Child (Chic). 2006 May-Aug;73(2):105-11.

Associations between a history of breast feeding, malocclusion and parafunctional habits in Puerto Rican children.

López Del Valle LM, Singh GD, Feliciano N, Machuca Mdel C. P R Health Sci J. 2006 Mar;25(1):31-4.

Breast-feeding and deleterious oral habits in mouth and nose breathers. Trawitzki LV, Anselmo-Lima WT, Melchior MO, Grechi TH, Valera FC. Braz J Otorhinolaryngol. 2005 Nov-Dec;71(6):747-51.

Changes in the prevalence of nonnutritive sucking patterns in the first 8 years of life. Bishara SE, Warren JJ, Broffitt B, Levy SM. Am J Orthod Dentofacial Orthop. 2006 Jul;130(1):31-6.

Association between allergic rhinitis, bottle feeding, non-nutritive sucking habits, and malocclusion in the primary dentition. Vázquez-Nava F, Quezada-Castillo JA, Oviedo-Treviño S, Saldivar-González AH, Sánchez-Nuncio HR, Beltrán-Guzmán FJ, Vázquez-Rodríguez EM, Vázquez Rodríguez CF. Arch Dis Child. 2006 Oct;91(10):836-40. Epub 2006 Jun 12.

Dental arch diameters and relationships to oral habits. Aznar T, Galán AF, Marín I, Domínguez A. Angle Orthod. 2006 May;76(3):441-5.

Effects of nonnutritive sucking habits on occlusal characteristics in the mixed dentition. Warren JJ, Slayton RL, Bishara SE, Levy SM, Yonezu T, Kanellis MJ. Pediatr Dent. 2005 Nov-Dec;27(6):445-50.

Predictors for Haemophilus influenzae colonization, antibiotic resistance and for sharing an identical isolate among children attending 16 licensed day-care centers in Michigan. Barbosa-Cesnik C, Farjo RS, Patel M, Gilsdorf J, McCoy SI, Pettigrew MM, Marrs C, Foxman B. Pediatr Infect Dis J. 2006 Mar;25(3):219-23.

[Presence of temporomandibular joint discomfort related to pacifier use]. Tosato Jde P, Biasotto-Gonzalez DA, Gonzalez Tde O. Braz J Otorhinolaryngol. 2005 May-Jun;71(3):365-8. Epub 2005 Dec 14. Portuguese.

Pattern and severity of early childhood caries. Hallett KB, O'Rourke PK. Community Dent Oral Epidemiol. 2006 Feb;34(1):25-35.

Feeding-facilitating techniques for the nursing infant with Robin sequence. Nassar E, Marques IL, Trindade AS Jr, Bettiol H. Cleft Palate Craniofac J. 2006 Jan;43(1):55-60.

[Removal of sucking habits and myofunctional therapy: establishing swallowing and tongue rest position].

Degan VV, Puppin-Rontani RM. Pro Fono. 2005 Apr-Dec;17(3):375-82. Portuguese.

[Etiological aspects of anterior open bite and its implications to the oral functions]. Maciel CT, Leite IC.

Pro Fono. 2005 Apr-Dec;17(3):293-302. Portuguese.

Unilateral posterior crossbite with mandibular shift: a review. Kennedy DB, Osepchook M. J Can Dent Assoc. 2005 Sep;71(8):569-73. Review.

A successful approach to the management of children: part 4. Berman MH. Dent Today. 2005 Aug;24(8):76-81.

Feeding, artificial sucking habits, and malocclusions in 3-year-old girls in different regions of the world. Caglar E, Larsson E, Andersson EM, Hauge MS, Ogaard B, Bishara S, Warren J, Noda T, Dolci GS. J Dent Child (Chic). 2005 Jan-Apr;72(1):25-30.

Feeding habits and severe early childhood caries in Brazilian preschool children. Azevedo TD, Bezerra AC, de Toledo OA. Pediatr Dent. 2005 Jan-Feb;27(1):28-33.

[Effect of the early intervention of oral habits on the development of dental occlusion]. Bertoldi PM, Felfício CM, Matsumoto MA. Pro Fono. 2005 Jan-Apr;17(1):37-44. Portuguese.

Oral health, sociodemographic factors, dietary and oral hygiene practices in Jordanian children. Sayegh A, Dini EL, Holt RD, Bedi R. J Dent. 2005 May;33(5):379-88. Epub 2004 Dec 13.

Pacifier sucking in a child with cleft palate: occlusal consequences. Romero M, Bravo LA, Romero P.

Cleft Palate Craniofac J. 2005 Mar;42(2):218-9.

Relationship between oral parafunctional/nutritive sucking habits and temporomandibular joint dysfunction in primary dentition. Castelo PM, Gavião MB, Pereira LJ, Bonjardim LR. Int J Paediatr Dent. 2005 Jan;15(1):29-36.

Prevalence of pacifier-sucking habits and successful methods to eliminate them--a preliminary study. Degan VV, Puppin-Rontani RM. J Dent Child (Chic). 2004 May-Aug;71(2):148-51.

[Feeding habits of breastfed and non-breastfed children up to 1 year old].Vieira GO, Silva LR, Vieira Tde O, Almeida JA, Cabral VA. J Pediatr (Rio J). 2004 Sep-Oct;80(5):411-6. Portuguese.

[The relationship between oral habits, oronasopharyngeal alterations, and malocclusion in preschool children in Vitória, Espírito Santo, Brazil]. Emmerich A, Fonseca L, Elias AM, de Medeiros UV. Cad Saude Publica. 2004 May-Jun;20(3):689-97. Epub 2004 May 19. Portuguese.

The behavior and routes of lead exposure in pregrasping infants. Kranz BD, Simon DL, Leonardi BG.

J Expo Anal Environ Epidemiol. 2004 Jul;14(4):300-11.

The digit sucking habit and related factors: observations from a child dental health clinic in Nigeria.

daCosta OO, Orenuga OO. Afr J Med Med Sci. 2003 Jun;32(2):167-71.

The effects of infant feeding patterns on the occlusion of the primary dentition. Charchut SW, Allred EN, Needleman HL. J Dent Child (Chic). 2003 Sep-Dec;70(3):197-203.

Prevalence of oral mucosal alterations in children from 0 to 12 years old. Bessa CF, Santos PJ, Aguiar MC, do Carmo MA. J Oral Pathol Med. 2004 Jan;33(1):17-22.

Cross-sectional study of oral mucosal conditions among a central Amazonian Indian community, Brazil.

dos Santos PJ, Bessa CF, de Aguiar MC, do Carmo MA. J Oral Pathol Med. 2004 Jan;33(1):7-12.

Pacifier use in children: a review of recent literature. Adair SM. Pediatr Dent. 2003 Sep-Oct;25(5):449-58. Review.

Malocclusion associated with abnormal posture. Yamaguchi H, Sueishi K. Bull Tokyo Dent Coll. 2003 May;44(2):43-54.

Effects of different pacifiers on the primary dentition and oral myofunctional strutures of preschool children.

Zardetto CG, Rodrigues CR, Stefani FM. Pediatr Dent. 2002 Nov-Dec;24(6):552-60.

Prevalence of malocclusion in 4-6-year-old Brazilian children. Chevitarese AB, Della Valle D, Moreira TC.

J Clin Pediatr Dent. 2002 Fall;27(1):81-5.

Caries prevalence and patterns and their relationship to social class, infant feeding and oral hygiene in 4-5-year-old children in Amman, Jordan. Sayegh A, Dini EL, Holt RD, Bedi R. Community Dent Health. 2002 Sep;19(3):144-51.

[Significance of bad habits in orthodontics]. Tarján I. Fogorv Sz. 2002 Aug;95(4):135-42. Review. Hungarian.

Associations of pacifier use, digit sucking, and child care attendance with cessation of breastfeeding. Levy SM, Slager SL, Warren JJ, Levy BT, Nowak AJ. J Fam Pract. 2002 May;51(5):465.

Duration of nutritive and nonnutritive sucking behaviors and their effects on the dental arches in the primary dentition. Warren JJ, Bishara SE. Am J Orthod Dentofacial Orthop. 2002 Apr;121(4):347-56.

Breastfeeding is early functional jaw orthopedics (an introduction). Page DC. Funct Orthod. 2001 Fall;18(3):24-7.

Relation of oral yeast infection in Brazilian infants and use of a pacifier. Mattos-Graner RO, de Moraes AB, Rontani RM, Birman EG. ASDC J Dent Child. 2001 Jan-Feb;68(1):33-6, 10.

Pacifier-sucking associated with a bizarre habit: a case report. Vieira AR, Modesto A. J Clin Pediatr Dent. 2000 Spring;24(3):187-9.

Sucking, chewing, and feeding habits and the development of crossbite: a longitudinal study of girls from birth to 3 years of age. Larsson E. Angle Orthod. 2001 Apr;71(2):116-9.

[Pacifier use: risks and benefits].Martínez Sánchez L, Díaz González E, García-Tornel Florensa S, Gaspà Martí J.

An Esp Pediatr. 2000 Dec;53(6):580-5. Review. Spanish.

Socio-demographic associations with digit and pacifier sucking at 15 months of age and possible associations with infant infection. The ALSPAC Study Team. Avon Longitudinal Study of Pregnancy and Childhood. North Stone K, Fleming P, Golding J. Early Hum Dev. 2000 Dec;60(2):137-48.

Provision of supplementary fluids to breast fed infants and later breast-feeding success. Kind C, Schubiger G, Schwarz U, Tönz O. Adv Exp Med Biol. 2000;478:347-54.

[The relationship between oral habits and malocclusion in preschool children]. Tomita NE, Bijella VT, Franco LJ.

Rev Saude Publica. 2000 Jun;34(3):299-303. Portuguese.

Non-nutritive sucking behaviors in preschool children: a longitudinal study. Warren JJ, Levy SM, Nowak AJ, Tang S. Pediatr Dent. 2000 May-Jun;22(3):187-91.

Association between early weaning, non-nutritive sucking habits and occlusal anomalies in 3-year-old Finnish children. Karjalainen S, Rönning O, Lapinleimu H, Simell O. Int J Paediatr Dent. 1999 Sep;9(3):169-73.

Urticaria and hidden salicylates. Wright AL, Minford A. Pediatr Dermatol. 1999 Nov-Dec;16(6):463-4.

Early nutrition, essential fatty acid status and visual acuity of term infants at 7 months of age. Bakker EC, van Houwelingen AC, Hornstra G. Eur J Clin Nutr. 1999 Nov;53(11):872-9.

Caries pattern and oral health habits in 2- to 6-year-old children exhibiting differing levels of caries. Gizani S, Vinckier F, Declerck D. Clin Oral Investig. 1999 Mar;3(1):35-40.

Breastfeeding patterns in relation to thumb sucking and pacifier use. Aarts C, Hörnell A, Kylberg E, Hofvander Y, Gebre-Medhin M. Pediatrics. 1999 Oct;104(4):e50.

Pacifier use and otitis media in infants twelve months of age or younger. Jackson JM, Mourino AP. Pediatr Dent. 1999 Jul-Aug;21(4):255-60.

Pacifier use and morbidity in the first six months of life. North K, Fleming P, Golding J. Pediatrics. 1999 Mar;103(3): E34.

An analysis of malocclusion in children with otitis media. Watase S, Mourino AP, Tipton GA. Pediatr Dent. 1998 Sep-Oct;20(5):327-30.

Profile of non-nutritive sucking habits in relation to nursing behavior in pre-school children. Vadiakas G, Oulis C, Berdouses E. J Clin Pediatr Dent. 1998 Winter;22(2):133-6.

Risk factors for colonization of salivary lactobacilli and Candida in children. Ollila P, Niemelä M, Uhari M, Larmas M. Acta Odontol Scand. 1997 Jan;55(1):9-13.

Nutritive and nonnutritive sucking habits: a review. Turgeon-O'Brien H, Lachapelle D, Gagnon PF, Larocque I, Maheu-Robert LF. ASDC J Dent Child. 1996 Sep-Oct;63(5):321-7. Review.

Effects of current and former pacifier use on the dentition of 24- to 59-month-old children. Adair SM, Milano M, Lorenzo I, Russell C. Pediatr Dent. 1995 Nov-Dec;17(7):437-44.

[What physicians should currently observe in the area of dental health]. Büttner M. Gesundheitswesen. 1995 Nov;57(11):741-3. German.

The epidemiology of sleep related breathing disorder in children. Hultcrantz E, Löfstrand-Tideström B, Ahlquist-Rastad J. Int J Pediatr Otorhinolaryngol. 1995 Jun;32 Suppl:S63-6.

Artificial sucking habits: etiology, prevalence and effect on occlusion. Larsson E. Int J Orofacial Myology. 1994 Nov;20:10-21.

The effect of sucking habits, cohort, sex, intercanine arch widths, and breast or bottle feeding on posterior crossbite in Norwegian and Swedish 3-year-old children. Øgaard B, Larsson E, Lindsten R. Am J Orthod Dentofacial Orthop. 1994 Aug;106(2):161-166.

The effect of sucking habits, cohort, sex, intercanine arch widths, and breast or bottle feeding on posterior crossbite in Norwegian and Swedish 3-year-old children. Ogaard B, Larsson E, Lindsten R. Am J Orthod Dentofacial Orthop. 1994 Aug;106(2):161-6.

Pacifiers and dental structure as risk factors for otitis media. Niemelä M, Uhari M, Hannuksela A. Int J Pediatr Otorhinolaryngol. 1994 Apr;29(2):121-7.

Evaluation of the change in the knowledge of community regarding infant dental care subsequent to intervention strategies through existing health manpower in rural areas of Haryana (India). Tewari A, Gauba K, Goyal A. J Indian Soc Pedod Prev Dent. 1994 Mar;12(1):29-34.

Release of preventive agents from pacifiers in vitro. An introduction to a novel preventive measure. Suhonen J, Sener B, Bucher W, Lutz F. Schweiz Monatsschr Zahnmed. 1994;104(8):946-51.

The effect of hypertrophic adenoids and tonsils on the development of posterior crossbite and oral habits. Oulis CJ, Vadiakas GP, Ekonomides J, Dratsa J. J Clin Pediatr Dent. 1994 Spring;18(3):197-201.

The Finnish Family Competence Study: the effects of living conditions on sucking habits in 3-year-old Finnish children and the association between these habits and dental occlusion. Paunio P, Rautava P, Sillanpää M. Acta Odontol Scand. 1993 Feb;51(1):23-9.

[The development of the deciduous dentition under the influence of differently shaped pacifiers]. Eismann D, Mender G. Fortschr Kieferorthop. 1992 Dec;53(6):349-53. German.

Evaluation of the effects of orthodontic pacifiers on the primary dentitions of 24- to 59-month-old children: preliminary study. Adair SM, Milano M, Dushku JC. Pediatr Dent. 1992 Jan-Feb;14(1):13-8.

Oral habits. A behavioral approach. Peterson JE Jr, Schneider PE. Pediatr Clin North Am. 1991 Oct;38(5):1289-307. Review.

Ill effects with use of pacifiers in children. Bhat IA, Shah GN, Hafeeza, Zahida. Indian J Matern Child Health. 1991;2(2):51-3.

Sucking habits: clinical management in dentistry. da Silva Filho OG, Gomes Gloncalves RJ, Maia FA. J Clin Pediatr Dent. 1991 Spring;15(3):137-56.

Non-nutritive suckling and use of pacifiers. Mathur GP, Mathur S, Khanduja GS. Indian Pediatr. 1990 ov;27(11):1187-9.

[Elimination of the pacifier habit]. Luque Coqui M. Pract Odontol. 1989 Feb;10(2):8, 10. Spanish.

Bottle-feeding and malocclusion: is there an association? Meyers A, Hertzberg J. Am J Orthod Dentofacial Orthop. 1988 Feb;93(2):149-52.

The thumb, the pacifier, the erupting tooth and a beautiful smile. Baer PN, Lester M. J Pedod. 1987 inter;11(2):113-9. No abstract available. Erratum in: J Pedod 1987 Summer;11(4):399.

Pacifiers: the positive side. Anderson GC. MCN Am J Matern Child Nurs. 1986 Mar-Apr;11(2):122-4. No abstract available.

[Influence of thumb sucking and pacifiers on deciduous teeth]. Schlömer R. Fortschr Kieferorthop. 1984 pr;45(2):141-8. German. No abstract available.

[The initial frequency of pacifier and fingersucking habits]. Larsson E. Tandlakartidningen. 1983 Jun 5;75(12):695-9. Swedish. No abstract available.

Amount of sucking when a sucking object is readily available to human newborns. Koepke JE, Barnes P. Child Dev. 1982 Aug;53(4):978-83.

Nursing habits and dental decay in infants: "nursing bottle caries". Ripa LW. ASDC J Dent Child. 1978 Jul- Aug;45(4):274-5.

[Pacifiers or thumbs]. Pfefferkorn M. Quintessenz J. 1977 May;7(5):27-8. German. No abstract available.

Thumb- and pacifier-sucking habits. Zadik D, Stern N, Litner M. Am J Orthod. 1977 Feb;71(2):197-201.

[The child and one of its substitute love object: the pacifier (author's transl)]. Akerman B. Ortodontia. 1975 Jan-Apr;8(1):29-37. Portuguese. No abstract available.

[Will the pacifier be used once again?]. Geller L. Osterr Hebammenztg. 1973 Jan;20(2):6-7. German. No abstract available.

[Relationship between fingersucking and the use of a pacifier]. Muñiz MA, De Muñiz BR. Rev Asoc Odontol Argent. 1970 Jul-Sep;58(7):95-100. Spanish.

Search Results Anterior Open Bite Treatment:

Posterior teeth angulation in non-extraction and extraction treatment of anterior open-bite patients. Janson G, Rizzo M, Laranjeira V, Garib DG, Valarelli FP. Prog Orthod. 2017 Dec;18(1):13.

Comparison of two treatment strategies for the early treatment of an anterior skeletal open bite: Posterior bite block-vertical pull chin cup (PBB-VPC) vs. posterior bite block-high pull headgear (PBB-HPH). Turkkahraman H, Cetin E. J Orofac Orthop. 2017 Jul;78(4):338-347.

Nonsurgical correction using miniscrew-assisted vertical control of a severe high angle with mandibular retrusion and gummy smile in an adult. Wang XD, Zhang JN, Liu DW, Lei FF, Liu WT, Song Y, Zhou YH. Am J Orthod Dentofacial Orthop. 2017 May;151(5):978-988

Nonsurgical treatment of severe Class II malocclusion with anterior open bite using mini-implants and maxillary lateral incisor and mandibular first molar extractions. Pithon MM. Am J Orthod Dentofacial Orthop. 2017 ay;151(5):964-977.

Nonsurgical Treatment of a Severe Skeletal Anterior Open Bite. Kassir C, Saade A. J Clin Orthod. 2017 Feb;51(2):103-112. No abstract available.

Camouflage of a high-angle skeletal Class II open-bite malocclusion in an adult after mini-implant failure during treatment. Franzotti Sant'Anna E, Carneiro da Cunha A, Paludo Brunetto D, Franzotti Sant'Anna C. Am J Orthod Dentofacial Orthop. 2017 Mar;151(3):583-597

Treatment of Anterior Open Bite with a Mini-Implant-Supported Tongue Crib. Kalia AJ. J Clin Orthod. 2017 Jan;51(1):37-45.

Are temporary anchorage devices truly effective in the treatment of skeletal open bites? Turkkahraman H, Sarioglu M. Eur J Dent. 2016 Oct-Dec;10(4):447-453.

[Etiology and treatment options of anterior open bite in growing patients: a narrative review]. Caprioglio A, Fastuca R. Orthod Fr. 2016 Dec;87(4):467-477. Epub 2016 Dec 12. Review. French.

[Retaining corrected skeletal open bites. How can we increase the stability of our results?] Littlewood SJ.

Orthod Fr. 2016 Dec;87(4):457-465. Epub 2016 Dec 12. French.

Retrospective study of maxillary sinus dimensions and pneumatization in adult patients with an anterior open bite.

Ryu J, Choi SH, Cha JY, Lee KJ, Hwang CJ. Am J Orthod Dentofacial Orthop. 2016 Nov;150(5):796-801

Nasal breathing and the vertical dimension: A cephalometric study. El Aouame A, Daoui A, El Quars F. Int Orthod. 2016 Dec;14(4):491-502.

Dimensional changes of dental arches produced by fixed and removable palatal cribs: A prospective, randomized, controlled study. Slaviero T, Fernandes TM, Oltramari-Navarro PV, de Castro AC, Conti F, Poleti ML, de Almeida MR. Angle Orthod. 2017 Mar;87(2):215-222.

Nonsurgical treatment of skeletal anterior open bite in adult patients: Posterior build-ups. Vela-Hernández A, López-García R, García-Sanz V, Paredes-Gallardo V, Lasagabaster-Latorre F. Angle Orthod. 2017 Jan;87(1):33-40.

Modified Occlusal Settling Appliance in Twin Block Therapy. Singh H, Maurya R, Kapoor P, Sharma P. J Clin Diagn Res. 2016 Sep;10(9): ZH01-ZH02.

Dentoskeletal effects produced by removable palatal crib, bonded spurs, and chincup therapy in growing children with anterior open bite. Insabralde NM, de Almeida RR, Henriques JF, Fernandes TM, Flores-Mir C, de Almeida MR. Angle Orthod. 2016 Nov;86(6):969-975.

Systematic review for orthodontic and orthopedic treatments for anterior open bite in the mixed dentition. Pisani L, Bonaccorso L, Fastuca R, Spena R, Lombardo L, Caprioglio A. Prog Orthod. 2016 Dec;17(1):28

Severe Anterior Open Bite during Mixed Dentition Treated with Palatal Spurs. Nascimento MH, de Araújo TM, Machado AW. J Clin Pediatr Dent. 2016;40(3):247-50.

Anterior Open Bite In 27 Months Old Children after Use of a Novel Pacifier - A Cohort Study. Zimmer S, Zuralski H, Bizhang M, Ostermann T, Barthel CR. J Clin Pediatr Dent. 2016;40(4):328-33.

Evaluation of long-term stability of skeletal anterior open bite correction in adults treated with maxillary posterior segment intrusion using zygomatic miniplates. Marzouk ES, Kassem HE. Am J Orthod Dentofacial Orthop. 2016 Jul;150(1):78-88.

Dilemmas in Treatment of Recurrent Recalcitrant Dental Anterior Open Bite. Palencar AJ. Int J Orthod Milwaukee. 2016 Spring;27(1):19-24.

Nonsurgical treatment of an adult with an open bite and large lower anterior facial height with edgewise appliances and temporary anchorage devices. Fukui T, Kano H, Saito I. Am J Orthod Dentofacial Orthop. 2016 Jun;149(6):889-98.

Anterior open-bite treatment with bonded vs conventional lingual spurs: A comparative study. Canuto LF, Janson G, de Lima NS, de Almeida RR, Cançado RH. Am J Orthod Dentofacial Orthop. 2016 Jun;149(6):847-55.

Skeletal and Dentoalveolar Cephalometric Features of Anterior Open Bite among Yemeni Adults. Daer AA, Abuaffan AH. Scientifica (Cairo). 2016; 2016:3147972.

Effect of a thin-neck pacifier on primary dentition: a randomized controlled trial. Wagner Y, Heinrich-Weltzien R.

Orthod Craniofac Res. 2016 Aug;19(3):127-36.

Comparisons of two protocols for early treatment of anterior open bite. Mucedero M, Vitale M, Franchi L, Cozza P, Perillo L. Eur J Orthod. 2016 May 3:270-276

Anterior open-bite orthodontic treatment in an adult patient: A clinical case report. Gracco A, Siviero L, de Stefani A, Bruno G, Stellini E. Int Orthod. 2016 Jun;14(2):171-83.

Effects of simultaneous palatal expansion and mandibular advancement in a child suffering from OSA. Galeotti A, Festa P, Pavone M, De Vincentiis GC. Acta Otorhinolaryngol Ital. 2016 Aug;36(4):328-332.

Closure of an open bite using the 'Mousetrap' appliance: a 3-year follow-up. Wilmes B, Vasudavan S, Stocker B, Willmann JH, Drescher D. Aust Orthod J. 2015 Nov;31(2):208-15.

Effect of molar intrusion with temporary anchorage devices in patients with anterior open bite: a systematic review.

Alsafadi AS, Alabdullah MM, Saltaji H, Abdo A, Youssef M. Prog Orthod. 2016; 17:9.

Prevalence of occlusal traits and orthodontic treatment need in 14-year-old adolescents in Northeast Italy. Ferro R, Besostri A, Olivieri A, Stellini E. Eur J Paediatr Dent. 2016 Mar;17(1):36-42.

Cephalometric configuration of the occlusal plane in patients with anterior open bite. Choi YJ, Kim DJ, Nam J, Chung CJ, Kim KH. Am J Orthod Dentofacial Orthop. 2016 Mar;149(3):391-400

Effectiveness of open bite correction when managing deleterious oral habits in growing children and adolescents: a systematic review and meta-analysis. Feres MF, Abreu LG, Insabralde NM, de Almeida MR, Flores-Mir C. Eur J Orthod. 2017 Feb;39(1):31-42.

Open-bite treatment with vertical control and tongue reeducation. Garrett J, Araujo E, Baker C. Am J Orthod Dentofacial Orthop. 2016 Feb;149(2):269-76.

Effects of palatal crib and bonded spurs in early treatment of anterior open bite: A prospective randomized clinical study. Leite JS,

Matiussi LB, Salem AC, Provenzano MG, Ramos AL. Angle Orthod. 2016 Sep;86(5):734-9.

Giving back to our specialty: Participate in the national anterior open-bite study. Huang GJ. Am J Orthod Dentofacial Orthop. 2016 Jan;149(1):4-5.

Intraoral Vertical Ramus Osteotomy Results in Good Long-Term Mandibular Stability in Patients with Mandibular Prognathism and Anterior Open Bite. Choi SH, Cha JY, Park HS, Hwang CJ. J Oral Maxillofac Surg. 2016 Apr;74(4):804-10.

Influence of maxillary posterior discrepancy on upper molar vertical position and facial vertical dimensions in subjects with or without skeletal open bite. Arriola-Guillén LE, Aliaga-Del Castillo A, Pérez-Vargas LF, Flores-Mir C. Eur J Orthod. 2016 Jun;38(3):251-8

Molar Intrusion in Open-bite Adults Using Zygomatic Miniplates. Marzouk ES, Abdallah EM, El-Kenany WA.

Int J Orthod Milwaukee. 2015 Summer;26(2):47-54.

[Lingual treatment of an anterior open bite case]. Gallardo R. Orthod Fr. 2015 Jun;86(2):151-60.

Influence of non-orthodontic intervention on digit sucking and consequent anterior open bite: a preliminary study.

Huang B, Lejarraga C, Franco CS, Kang Y, Lee A, Abbott J, Takahashi K, Bessho K, Pumtang-on P. Int Dent J. 2015 Oct;65(5):235-41

Mini-implant-anchored Mesialslider for simultaneous mesialisation and intrusion of upper molars in an anterior open bite case: a three-year follow-up. Wilmes B, Katyal V, Willmann J, Stocker B, Drescher D. Aust Orthod J. 2015 May;31(1):87-97.

Innovation in prediction planning for anterior open bite correction. Almuzian M, Almukhtar A, O'Neil M, Benington P, Al Anezi T, Ayoub A. Aust Orthod J. 2015 May;31(1):78-86.

Changes of some functional speech disorders after surgical correction of skeletal anterior open bite. Knez Ambrožič M, Hočevar Boltežar I, Ihan Hren N. Int J Rehabil Res. 2015 Sep;38(3):246-52.

Prevalence of dyslalias in 8 to 16-year-old students with anterior open bite in the municipality of Envigado, Colombia. Ocampo-Parra A, Escobar-Toro B, Sierra-Alzate V, Rueda ZV, Lema MC. BMC Oral Health. 2015 Jul 10; 15:77.

An Aesthetic and Functional Rehabilitation: A Case Study. Ali J, Calamia C, Magid KS, Calamia JR, Giannuzzi NJ.

Dent Clin North Am. 2015 Jul;59(3):547-57

Effectiveness of the open bite treatment in growing children and adolescents. A systematic review. Feres MF, Abreu LG, Insabralde NM, Almeida MR, Flores-Mir C. Eur J Orthod. 2016 Jun;38(3):237-50.

The effect of orofacial myofunctional treatment in children with anterior open bite and tongue dysfunction: a pilot study. Van Dyck C, Dekeyser A, Vantricht E, Manders E, Goeleven A, Fieuws S, Willems G. Eur J Orthod. 2016 Jun;38(3):227-34.

Anterior open bite treated with myofunctional therapy and palatal crib. Asiry MA. J Contemp Dent Pract. 2015 Mar 1;16(3):243-7.

Geometry of anterior open bite correction. Abramson ZR, Susarla SM, Lawler ME, Choudhri AF, Peacock ZS.

J Craniofac Surg. 2015 May;26(3): e223-5.

Morphology of open bite. Krey KF, Dannhauer KH, Hierl T. J Orofac Orthop. 2015 May;76(3):213-24.

Anterior open bite--simplified non-surgical technique to correct in adults. Jefferson Y. Int J Orthod Milwaukee. 2015 Spring;26(1):19-24.

Prevalence and change of malocclusions from primary to early permanent dentition: a longitudinal study. Dimberg L, Lennartsson B, Arnrup K, Bondemark L. Angle Orthod. 2015 Sep;85(5):728-34

Nonsurgical approach to Class I open-bite malocclusion with extrusion mechanics: a 3-year retention case report.

Atsawasuwan P, Hohlt W, Evans CA. Am J Orthod Dentofacial Orthop. 2015 Apr;147(4):499-508.

Interventions for the cessation of non-nutritive sucking habits in children. Borrie FR, Bearn DR, Innes NP, Iheozor-Ejiofor Z. Cochrane Database Syst Rev. 2015 Mar 31;(3):CD008694.

Orthodontic Treatment of Skeletal Class II Adolescent with Anterior Open Bite using Mini-Screws and Modified Palatal Anchorage Plate. Kook YA, Park JH, Kim Y, Ahn CS, Bayome M. J Clin Pediatr Dent. 2015 Winter;39(2):187-92.

Evaluating the Stability of Open Bite Treatments and Its Predictive Factors in the Retention Phase during Permanent Dentition. Salehi P, Pakshir HR, Hoseini SA. J Dent (Shiraz). 2015 Mar;16(1):22-9.

Biomechanical considerations in the correction of anterior open bite with maxillary skeletal plates. Jack Burrow S 3rd. J Clin Orthod. 2015 Jan;49(1):35-45.

Orthognathic correction of dento-facial discrepancies. Cunningham SJ, Johal A. Br Dent J. 2015 Feb 16;218(3):167-75.

Multidisciplinary correction of anterior open bite relapse and upper airway obstruction. Gracco A, Perri A, Siviero L, Bonetti GA, Cocilovo F, Stellini E. Korean J Orthod. 2015 Jan;45(1):47-56.

Early treatment of anterior open bite: Comparison of the vertical and horizontal morphological changes induced by magnetic bite-blocks and adjusted rapid molar intruders. Albogha MH, Takahashi I, Sawan MN. Korean J Orthod. 2015 Jan;45(1):38-46.

Occlusal characteristics of children with hypertrophied adenoids in Nigeria. Osiatuma VI, Otuyemi OD, Kolawole KA, Ogunbanjo BO, Amusa YB. Int Orthod. 2015 Mar;13(1):26-42.

Severity and outcome assessments of patients undertaking surgical orthodontic treatment. Zhao Y, Fowler PV.

Aust Orthod J. 2014 Nov;30(2):184-91.

Dentoskeletal changes following mini-implant molar intrusion in anterior open bite patients. Hart TR, Cousley RR, Fishman LS, Tallents RH. Angle Orthod. 2015 Nov;85(6):941-8.

Prevalence of malocclusion and orthodontic treatment needs among 12-15-year-old school children of fishermen of Kutch coast, Gujarat, India. Sanadhya S, Chadha M, Chaturvedi MK, Chaudhary M, Lerra S, Meena MK, Bakutra G, Acharya S, Pandey A, Tak M, Asawa K, Kamate S. Int Marit Health. 2014;65(3):106-13.

Cephalometric study of the upper airways and dentoalveolar height in open bite patients. Laranjo F, Pinho T.

Int Orthod. 2014 Dec;12(4):467-82.

Severe anterior open bite with mandibular retrusion treated with multiloop edgewise archwires and microimplant anchorage complemented by genioplasty. Xu Z, Hu Z, Wang X, Shen G. Am J Orthod Dentofacial Orthop. 2014 Nov;146(5):655-64.

Outcomes and stability in patients with anterior open bite and long anterior face height treated with temporary anchorage devices and a maxillary intrusion splint. Scheffler NR, Proffit WR, Phillips C. Am J Orthod Dentofacial Orthop. 2014 Nov;146(5):594-602.

Orthodontic treatment of severe anterior open bite and alveolar bone defect complicated by an ankylosed maxillary central incisor: a case report. Lin F, Sun H, Yao L, Chen Q, Ni Z. Head Face Med. 2014 Nov 21;10:47.

The prevalence of malocclusion and oral habits among 5-7-year-old children. Kasparaviciene K, Sidlauskas A, Zasciurinskiene E, Vasiliauskas A, Juodzbalys G, Sidlauskas M, Marmaite U. Med Sci Monit. 2014 Oct 24; 20:2036-42.

The short-term skeleto-dental effects of a new spring for the intrusion of maxillary posterior teeth in open bite patients. Foot R, Dalci O, Gonzales C, Tarraf NE, Darendeliler MA. Prog Orthod. 2014 Sep 25; 15:56.

Orthodontic and orthopaedic treatment for anterior open bite in children. Lentini-Oliveira DA, Carvalho FR, Rodrigues CG, Ye Q,

Prado LB, Prado GF, Hu R. Cochrane Database Syst Rev. 2014 Sep 24;(9):CD005515.

Conservative orthodontic treatment for skeletal open bite associated with amelogenesis imperfecta. Bechor N, Finkelstein T, Shapira Y, Shpack N. J Dent Child (Chic). 2014 May-Aug;81(2):96-102.

Molar intrusion in the management of anterior openbite and 'high angle' Class II malocclusions. Cousley RR.

J Orthod. 2014 Sep;41 Suppl 1: S39-46.

Treatment and retention of relapsed anterior open-bite with low tongue posture and tongue-tie: A 10-year follow-up.

Seo YJ, Kim SJ, Munkhshur J, Chung KR, Ngan P, Kim SH. Korean J Orthod. 2014 Jul;44(4):203-16.

Long-term stability of anterior open bite correction in mixed dentition with a new treatment protocol. Celli D, Manente A, DeCarlo A, Deli R. Eur J Paediatr Dent. 2014 Jun;15(2):158-62.

Maxillary molar intrusion with zygomatic anchorage in open bite treatment: lateral and oblique cephalometric evaluation. Oliveira TF, Nakao CY, Gonçalves JR, Santos-Pinto A. Oral Maxillofac Surg. 2015 Mar;19(1):71-7.

Amelogenesis imperfecta and anterior open bite: Etiological, classification, clinical and management interrelationships. Alachioti XS, Dimopoulou E, Vlasakidou A, Athanasiou AE. J Orthod Sci. 2014 Jan;3(1):1-6.

Factors related to stability following the surgical correction of skeletal open bite. Ito G, Koh M, Fujita T, Shirakura M, Ueda H, Tanne K. Aust Orthod J. 2014 May;30(1):61-6.

Relapse of skeletal class III with anterior open bite after bimaxillary orthognathic surgery depending on maxillary posterior impaction and mandibular counterclockwise rotation. Kor HS, Yang HJ, Hwang SJ. J Craniomaxillofac Surg. 2014 Jul;42(5): e230-8.

Conservative treatment for a growing patient with a severe, developing skeletal Class III malocclusion and open bite. Xu Y, Zhu

P, Le L, Cai B. Am J Orthod Dentofacial Orthop. 2014 Jun;145(6):807-16.

Miniscrew-supported posterior intrusion for treatment of anterior open bite. Scheffler NR, Proffit WR. J Clin Orthod. 2014 Mar;48(3):158-68.

Dental and skeletal components of Class II open bite treatment with a modified Thurow appliance. Jacob HB, dos Santos-Pinto A, Buschang PH. Dental Press J Orthod. 2014 Jan-Feb;19(1):19-25.

Stability of anterior open bite correction of adults treated with lingual appliances. Pithon MM. Eur J Orthod. 2014 Apr;36(2):243.

Modified quad helix appliance for thumb sucking and cross bite correction. Vinay C, Sandeep V, Hanumanth Rao CH, Uloopi KS, Kumar AS. Contemp Clin Dent. 2013 Oct;4(4):523-6.

The impact of spur therapy in dentoalveolar open bite. Meyer-Marcotty P, Kochel J, Stellzig-Eisenhauer A.

Aust Orthod J. 2013 Nov;29(2):145-52.

Orthodontic-surgical treatment: neuromuscular evaluation in open and deep skeletal bite patients. Farronato G, Giannini L, Galbiati G, Stabilini SA, Maspero C. Prog Orthod. 2013 Oct 29; 14:41.

Does orthodontic treatment provide a real functional improvement? A case control study. Masci C, Ciarrocchi I, Spadaro A, Necozione S, Marci MC, Monaco A. BMC Oral Health. 2013 Oct 24; 13:57.

Treatment and retreatment of a patient with a severe anterior open bite. Bosio JA, Justus R. Am J Orthod Dentofacial Orthop. 2013 Oct;144(4):594-606.

Orthodontic treatment of anterior open bite: a review article--is surgery always necessary? Reichert I, Figel P, Winchester L. Oral Maxillofac Surg. 2014 Sep;18(3):271-7.

Angle Class I malocclusion with anterior open bite treated with extraction of permanent teeth. Pithon MM.

Dental Press J Orthod. 2013 Mar-Apr;18(2):133-40.

Magical NiTi expander. Katti CG, Katti G, Kallur R, Ghali SR. BMJ Case Rep. 2013 Jul 17;2013.

Evaluations of sagittal and vertical changes induced by surgically assisted rapid palatal expansion. Iodice G, Bocchino T, Casadei M, Baldi D, Robiony M. J Craniofac Surg. 2013 Jul;24(4):1210-4.

Multidisciplinary management of a child with severe open bite and amelogenesis imperfecta. Millet C, Duprez JP.

J Contemp Dent Pract. 2013 Mar 1;14(2):320-6.

Glossectomy as an adjunct to correct an open-bite malocclusion with shortened maxillary central incisor roots.

Tanaka OM, Guariza-Filho O, Carlini JL, Oliveira DD, Pithon MM, Camargo ES. Am J Orthod Dentofacial Orthop. 2013 Jul;144(1):130-40.

Treatment of anterior open bite and multiple missing teeth with lingual fixed appliances, double jaw surgery, and dental implants. Jung MH, Baik UB, Ahn SJ. Am J Orthod Dentofacial Orthop. 2013 Apr;143(4 Suppl):S125-36.

Combining traditional techniques to correct anterior open bite and posterior crossbite. Menezes LM, Ritter DE, Locks A. Am J Orthod Dentofacial Orthop. 2013 Mar;143(3):412-20.

The segmented arch approach: a method for orthodontic treatment of a severe Class III open-bite malocclusion.

Espinar-Escalona E, Barrera-Mora JM, Llamas-Carreras JM, Ruiz-Navarro MB. Am J Orthod Dentofacial Orthop. 2013 Feb;143(2):254-65.

Open bite treatment using clear aligners. Guarneri MP, Oliverio T, Silvestre I, Lombardo L, Siciliani G.

Angle Orthod. 2013 Sep;83(5):913-9.

Treatment of class II malocclusion with open bite and absence of central maxillary incisor lost by trauma aided by use of orthodontic mini-implants. Pithon MM. Dent Traumatol. 2014 Feb;30(1):65-70.

Stability after maxillary segmentation for correction of anterior open bite: a cohort study of 33 cases. Silva I, Suska F, Cardemil C, Rasmusson L. J Craniomaxillofac Surg. 2013 Oct;41(7): e154-8.

Open bite as a risk factor for orthodontic root resorption. Motokawa M, Terao A, Kaku M, Kawata T, Gonzales C, Darendeliler MA, Tanne K. Eur J Orthod. 2013 Dec;35(6):790-5.

Bonded spurs with high-pull chincup therapy for anterior open bite. Karthickeyan SS. Am J Orthod Dentofacial Orthop. 2013 Jan;143(1):2.

Long-term stability of anterior open-bite closure with bilateral sagittal split osteotomy. Fontes AM, Joondeph DR, Bloomquist DS, Greenlee GM, Wallen TR, Huang GJ. Am J Orthod Dentofacial Orthop. 2012 Dec;142(6):792-800.

Surgical-orthodontic treatment for skeletal class II malocclusion with vertical maxillary excess, anterior open bite, and transverse maxillary deficiency. Choi SH, Cha JY, Kang DY, Hwang CJ. J Craniofac Surg. 2012 Nov;23(6): e531-5.

Dentoalveolar comparative study between removable and fixed cribs, associated to chincup, in anterior open bite treatment. Torres FC, Almeida RR, Almeida-Pedrin RR, Pedrin F, Paranhos LR. J Appl Oral Sci. 2012 Sep-Oct;20(5):531-7.

A simplified approach to true molar intrusion. Flieger S, Ziebura T, Kleinheinz J, Wiechmann D. Head Face Med. 2012 Nov 7;8:30.

Tongue reduction for macroglossia in Beckwith Wiedemann syndrome: review and application of new technique.

Heggie AA, Vujcich NJ, Portnof JE, Morgan AT. Int J Oral Maxillofac Surg. 2013 Feb;42(2):185-91.

Prevalence of malocclusions and orthodontic treatment need in 8- to 12-year-old schoolchildren in Casablanca, Morocco. Bourzgui F, Sebbar M, Hamza M, Lazrak L, Abidine Z, El Quars F. Prog Orthod. 2012 Sep;13(2):164-72.

Skeletal Class III and anterior open bite treatment with different retention protocols: a report of three cases. Farret MM, Farret MM, Farret AM. J Orthod. 2012 Sep;39(3):212-23.

Closure of anterior open bites with mandibular surgery: advantages and disadvantages of this approach. Van Sickels JE, Wallender A. Oral Maxillofac Surg. 2012 Dec;16(4):361-7.

Anterior open bite correction using bite block: A case report. de Barros RT, Câmara PP, Aloise AC, Siqueira DF, Paranhos LR, Torres FC. Int J Orthod Milwaukee. 2012 Summer;23(2):11-5.

Stability of anterior open bite correction of adults treated with lingual appliances. Geron S, Wasserstein A, Geron Z.

Eur J Orthod. 2013 Oct;35(5):599-603.

Myths that persist about orofacial myology. Mason RM. Int J Orofacial Myology. 2011 Nov;37:26-38.

Partial glossectomy as an auxiliary method to orthodontic treatment of dentofacial deformity. Salmen FS, Dedivitis RA. Int Arch Otorhinolaryngol. 2012 Jul;16(3):414-7.

Combined orthodontic and orthognathic surgical treatment for the correction of skeletal anterior open-bite malocclusion: a systematic review on vertical stability. Solano-Hernández B, Antonarakis GS, Scolozzi P, Kiliaridis S. J Oral Maxillofac Surg. 2013 Jan;71(1):98-109.

Oral myiasis in children. Reddy MH, Das N, Vivekananda MR. Contemp Clin Dent. 2012 Apr;3(Suppl 1):S19-22.

Treatment of severe skeletal open bite deformity in patients with Möbius syndrome: a report of 3 cases. Cai M, Shen G, Fang B, Zhu M, Mao LX. J Oral Maxillofac Surg. 2012 Jun;70(6):e389-99.

Prevalence of dental features that indicate a need for early orthodontic treatment. Shalish M, Gal A, Brin I, Zini A, Ben-Bassat Y. Eur J Orthod. 2013 Aug;35(4):454-9.

Eight-year stability of a severe skeletal anterior open bite with a hyperdivergent growth pattern treated with an edgewise appliance and chin cup therapy. Cerci V, Cerci BB, Meira TM, Cerci DX, Tanaka OM. Am J Orthod Dentofacial Orthop. 2012 Apr;141(4):e65-74.

The application of skeletal anchorage in the correction of anterior open bite and skeletal Class III malocclusion: a paradigm shift. Tarraf NE. Ann R Australas Coll Dent Surg. 2012 Apr;21:113-9.

[Passive correction of an anterior open bite related to non-nutritive sucking habits: report of a case]. Ngom PI, Fall AT, Toure KO, Badiane A, Diouf JS, Ba KD. Odontostomatol Trop. 2011 Dec;34(136):5-10.

Versatility and benefits of mini-implants for vertical and sagittal anchorage in a growing open bite class II patient.

Estelita S, Janson G, Chiqueto K. J Orthod. 2012 Mar;39(1):43-53.

Changes in malocclusion over time in New Zealand adolescents. Page LA, Thomson WM, Quick AN. Aust Orthod J. 2011 Nov;27(2):169-75.

Stability of the miniplate osteosynthesis used for sagittal split osteotomy for closing an anterior open bite: an experimental study in mini-pigs. Nieblerová J, Foltán R, Hanzelka T, Pavlíková G, Vlk M, Klíma K, Samsonyan L.

Int J Oral Maxillofac Surg. 2012 Apr;41(4):482-8.

Anterior open bite: aetiology and management. Sandler PJ, Madahar AK, Murray A. Dent Update. 2011 Oct;38(8):522-4, 527-8, 531-2.

Pharyngeal airway space and frontal and sphenoid sinus changes after maxillomandibular advancement with counterclockwise rotation for Class II anterior open bite malocclusions. Prado FB, Rossi AC, Freire AR, Groppo FC, De Moraes M, Caria PH. Dentomaxillofac Radiol. 2012 Feb;41(2):103-9.

Perceptions of dental aesthetics of Class III and anterior open bite malocclusions: a comparison between 10- to 11-year-old schoolchildren and orthodontists. Hamdan AM, Singh V, Rock W. Angle Orthod. 2012 Mar;82(2):202-8

Effects of maxillary molar intrusion with zygomatic anchorage on the stomatognathic system in anterior open bite patients. Akan S, Kocadereli I, Aktas A, Taşar F. Eur J Orthod. 2013 Feb;35(1):93-102.

Orthodontic management of an originally surgically planned treatment of an open bite: a case report. Kassir C, Assi SB. Orthodontics (Chic.). 2011 Spring;12(1):60-9.

Nonsurgical treatment of an adult with severe anterior open bite. Jaiswal AK, Dua AK, Ranganathan LK, ascarenhas R, Gandhi S. J Clin Orthod. 2011 Jun;45(6):341-7; quiz 340.

Gender influence on occlusal characteristics of primary dentition in 4- to 6-year-old children of Bagalkot City, India.

Bhayya DP, Shyagali TR. Oral Health Prev Dent. 2011;9(1):17-27.

Orthodontic treatment of an anterior openbite with the aid of corticotomy procedure: Case report. Aljhani AS, Aldrees AM. Saudi Dent J. 2011 Apr;23(2):99-106.

Efficacy of a novel pacifier in the prevention of anterior open bite. Zimmer S, Barthel CR, Ljubicic R, Bizhang M, Raab WH. Pediatr Dent. 2011 Jan-Feb;33(1):52-5.

Smile esthetics: a methodology for success in a complex case. Paris JC, Ortet S, Larmy A, Brouillet JL, Faucher AJ.

Eur J Esthet Dent. 2011 Spring;6(1):50-74.

Treatment of Class II open bite complicated by an ankylosed maxillary central incisor. Hwang DH, Park KH, Kwon YD, Kim SJ. Angle Orthod. 2011 Jul;81(4):726-35.

[Open bite and and therapeutic strategy]. Halimi A, Zaoui F. Odontostomatol Trop. 2010 Sep;33(131):35-48. French.

Dental appliances with inadequate occlusal coverage: a case report. Chate RA, Falconer DT. Br Dent J. 2011 Feb 12;210(3):109-10.

Stability of treatment for anterior open-bite malocclusion: a meta-analysis. Greenlee GM, Huang GJ, Chen SS, Chen J, Koepsell T, Hujoel P. Am J Orthod Dentofacial Orthop. 2011 Feb;139(2):154-69.

Long-term stability of anterior open bite closure corrected by surgical-orthodontic treatment.

Teittinen M, Tuovinen V, Tammela L, Schätzle M, Peltomäki T. Eur J Orthod. 2012 Apr;34(2):238-43.

Management of an Adult with Spaced Dentition, Class III Malocclusion and Open-bite Tendency.

Kaya D, Taner TU. Eur J Dent. 2011 Jan;5(1):121-9.

A Surgery-first approach in surgical-orthodontic treatment of mandibular prognathism--a case report. Yu CC, Chen PH, Liou EJ, Huang CS, Chen YR. Chang Gung Med J. 2010 Nov-Dec;33(6):699-705.

Success rate of anterior open-bite orthodontic-orthognathic surgical treatment. Jensen U, Ruf S. Am J Orthod Dentofacial Orthop. 2010 Dec;138(6):716-9.

Treatment of anterior open bite with the Invisalign system. Schupp W, Haubrich J, Neumann I.J Clin Orthod. 2010 Aug;44(8):501-7.

Long-term stability of anterior open-bite treatment by intrusion of maxillary posterior teeth. Baek MS, Choi YJ, Yu HS, Lee KJ, Kwak J, Park YC. Am J Orthod Dentofacial Orthop. 2010 Oct;138(4):396.e1-9; discussion 396-8.

Interdisciplinary treatment of a patient with amelogenesis imperfecta, a skeletal Class III relationship, and an anterior open bite. Marşan G, Aksu IS, Kurt H, Kuvat SV, Cura N. World J Orthod. 2010 Fall;11(3):284-90.

Orthodontic treatment of a complex open-bite malocclusion with temporary anchorage devices: a case report.

Waldman AB. J Calif Dent Assoc. 2010 Aug;38(8):591-600.

Skeletal Class III and open bite treated with bilateral sagittal split osteotomy and molar intrusion using titanium screws. Togawa R, Iino S, Miyawaki S. Angle Orthod. 2010 Nov;80(6):1176-84.

Multiloop edgewise archwire in the treatment of a patient with an anterior open bite and a long face. Ribeiro GL, Regis S Jr, da Cunha

Tde M, Sabatoski MA, Guariza-Filho O, Tanaka OM. Am J Orthod Dentofacial Orthop. 2010 Jul;138(1):89-95.

Stability of anterior open-bite treatment with occlusal adjustment. Janson G, Crepaldi MV, Freitas KM, de Freitas MR, Janson W. Am J Orthod Dentofacial Orthop. 2010 Jul;138(1):14.e1-7; discussion 14-5.

Virtual restoration of anatomic jaw relationship to obtain a precise 3D model for total joint prosthesis construction for treatment of TMJ ankylosis with open bite. Zizelmann C, Bucher P, Rohner D, Gellrich NC, Kokemueller H, Hammer B. Int J Oral Maxillofac Surg. 2010 Oct;39(10):1012-5.

The occlusal effects of digit sucking habits amongst school children in Northamptonshire (UK). Mistry P, Moles DR, O'Neill J, Noar J. J Orthod. 2010 Jun;37(2):87-92.

A new type of modified Essix Retainer for anterior open bite retention. Uzdil F, Kayalioglu M, Kendi E, Toroglu MS. Prog Orthod. 2010;11(1):45-52.

Management of anterior open bite and retention using the Bluegrass Hawley retainer. Sethusa MP. SADJ. 2010 Apr;65(3):112, 114-6.

Relapse of anterior open bites treated with orthodontic appliances with and without orofacial myofunctional therapy.

Smithpeter J, Covell D Jr. Am J Orthod Dentofacial Orthop. 2010 May;137(5):605-14.

Management of severe anterior open-bite in an adult patient using miniscrews as skeletal anchorage. Rachala MR, Harikrishnan P. Int J Orthod Milwaukee. 2010 Spring;21(1):9-14.

Correction of anterior open bite using maxillary third molar anchorage. Uribe F, Posada L, Nanda R. J Clin Orthod. 2009 Dec;43(12):773-8.

A single appliance for the correction of digit-sucking, tongue-thrust, and posterior cross bite. Kulkarni GV, Lau D.

Pediatr Dent. 2010 Jan-Feb;32(1):61-3.

Orthodontic treatment of anterior open-bite malocclusion: stability 10 years postretention. Zuroff JP, Chen SH, Shapiro PA, Little RM, Joondeph DR, Huang GJ. Am J Orthod Dentofacial Orthop. 2010 Mar;137(3):302.e1-8; discussion 302-3.

Correction of skeletal Class II--anterior deep bite and prominent chin by forced surgical rotation of the mandible.

Mommaerts MY, López-Arcas JM, Schurmans AM. Br J Oral Maxillofac Surg. 2010 Jul;48(5):349-51.

A maxillary expander for treatment of unilateral posterior crossbite with anterior open bite. Aggarwal A, Nandakishore P, Nayak US. J Clin Orthod. 2009 Oct;43(10):655-63. No abstract available.

Long-term impact of tongue reduction on speech intelligibility, articulation and oromyofunctional behaviour in a child with Beckwith-Wiedemann syndrome. Van Lierde KM, Mortier G, Huysman E, Vermeersch H. Int J Pediatr Otorhinolaryngol. 2010 Mar;74(3):309-18.

Muscular response to functional treatment of skeletal open-bite and deep-bite cases: an electromyographic study.

Uslu O, Arat ZM, Beyazoya M, Taskiran OO. World J Orthod. 2010 Winter;11(4):e85-93.

Stability of open bite correction with sagittal split osteotomy and closing rotation of the mandible.

Stansbury CD, Evans CA, Miloro M, BeGole EA, Morris DE. J Oral Maxillofac Surg. 2010 Jan;68(1):149-59.

An unusual type of sucking habit in a patient with cleft lip and palate. Satyaprasad S. J Indian Soc Pedod Prev Dent. 2009 Oct-Dec;27(4):260-2.

The effect of posterior bite-plane on dentoskeletal changes in skeletal open-bite malocclusion. Meibodi SE, Fatahi Meybodi S, Samadi AH. J Indian Soc Pedod Prev Dent. 2009 Oct-Dec;27(4):202-4.

The use of bonded acrylic expander in patient with open-bite and oral breathing. Giancotti A, Greco M. Eur J Paediatr Dent. 2008 Dec;9(4 Suppl):3-8.

Maximizing tissue response in selected subjects with anterior open bites. Mostafa YA, El-Mangoury NH, Abou-El-Ezz AM, Heider AM. World J Orthod. 2009 Fall;10(3):187-95.

[Occlusal plane orientation and postoperative anterior open bite relapse]. Olivi P, Cheynet F, Chossegros C, Blanc JL. Rev Stomatol Chir Maxillofac. 2009 Nov;110(5):269-72.

Closure of the anterior open bite using mandibular sagittal split osteotomy. Bisase B, Johnson P, Stacey M. Br J Oral Maxillofac Surg. 2010 Jul;48(5):352-5.

Speedy surgical orthodontic treatment with skeletal anchorage in adults--sagittal correction and open bite correction.

Chung KR, Mitsugi M, Lee BS, Kanno T, Lee W, Kim SH. J Oral Maxillofac Surg. 2009 Oct;67(10):2130-48.

Combined treatment of open bite - long-term evaluation and relapse factors. Wriedt S, Buhl V, Al-Nawas B, Wehrbein H. J Orofac Orthop. 2009 Jul;70(4):318-26.

Treatment of an anterior open bite with the multiloop archwire technique. Canavarro C, Cosendey VL, Capelli J Jr.

World J Orthod. 2009 Summer;10(2):104-10.

A retrospective and prospective view of orofacial myology. Mason RM. Int J Orofacial Myology. 2008 Nov;34:5-14.

Transverse dentoskeletal features of anterior open bite in the mixed dentition. Ballanti F, Franchi L, Cozza P.

Angle Orthod. 2009 Jul;79(4):615-20.

Non-surgical treatment of a Class II malocclusion with skeletal hyperdivergency and anterior open bite.

Rodriguez Flores JM. Int J Orthod Milwaukee. 2009 Spring;20(1):15-22.

Combined use of miniscrews and clear appliances for the treatment of bialveolar protrusion without conventional brackets. Choi NC, Park YC, Jo YM, Lee KJ. Am J Orthod Dentofacial Orthop. 2009 May;135(5):671-81.

Prosthetic treatment for severe open bite malocclusion and loss of several teeth. Shimizu H, Ozaki M, Takahashi Y.

N Y State Dent J. 2009 Jan;75(1):59-61.

Closure of severe skeletal anterior open bite with zygomatic anchorage. Seres L, Kocsis A. J Craniofac Surg. 2009 Mar;20(2):478-82.

Distribution of malocclusion types among thumb suckers seeking orthodontic treatment. Singh SP, Utreja A, Chawla HS. J Indian Soc Pedod Prev Dent. 2008;26 Suppl 3:S114-7.

Effects of maxillary second molar extraction on dentofacial morphology before and after anterior open-bite treatment: a cephalometric study. Kojima K, Endo T, Shimooka S. Odontology. 2009 Jan;97(1):43-50.

Maxillary expansion and stability in the orthodontic-surgical treatment of skeletal anterior open bites. Bianchi A, Amadori S, Pironi M, Marchetti C.Prog Orthod. 2009;10(2):26-37.

[Case report of an osteoarthritic temporomandibular joint patient whose posterior open bite was successfully restored by occlusal bonding method]. Minakuchi H. Nihon Hotetsu Shika Gakkai Zasshi. 2008 Oct;52(4):574-7.

Vertical control in nonextraction treatment of growing patients with anterior skeletal open bite. Spena R, Gracco A.

J Clin Orthod. 2008 Aug;42(8):443-9; quiz 455-6.

Non-surgical treatment of anterior open bite and its assessment using the Dawjee analysis: a case report. Dawjee SM, Oberholzer TG, Hlongwa P. SADJ. 2008 May;63(4):234, 236-8.

Three-year stability of open-bite correction by 1-piece maxillary osteotomy. Espeland L, Dowling PA, Mobarak KA, Stenvik A. Am J Orthod Dentofacial Orthop. 2008 Jul;134(1):60-6.

Evaluation of anterior open-bite treatment with occlusal adjustment. Janson G, Crepaldi MV, de Freitas KM, de Freitas MR, Janson W. Am J Orthod Dentofacial Orthop. 2008 Jul;134(1):10-1.

[Open-bite closure by intruding maxillary molars with skeletal anchorage]. Seres L, Kocsis A. Fogorv Sz. 2008 Feb;101(1):13-8.

Open bite correction by intrusion of posterior teeth with miniscrews. Park YC, Lee HA, Choi NC, Kim DH.

Angle Orthod. 2008 Jul;78(4):699-710.

A case of anterior open bite with severely narrowed maxillary dental arch and hypertrophic palatine tonsils.

Tanimoto K, Suzuki A, Nakatani Y, Yanagida T, Tanne Y, Tanaka E, Tanne K. J Orthod. 2008 Mar;35(1):5-15.

Orthodontic treatment of anterior open bite. Ng CS, Wong WK, Hagg U. Int J Paediatr Dent. 2008 Mar;18(2):78-83.

Treatment results and long-term stability of anterior open bite malocclusion. Remmers D, Van't Hullenaar RW, Bronkhorst EM, Bergé SJ, Katsaros C. Orthod Craniofac Res. 2008 Feb;11(1):32-42.

Skeletal Class III severe openbite treatment using implant anchorage. Sakai Y, Kuroda S, Murshid SA, Takano-Yamamoto T. Angle Orthod. 2008 Jan;78(1):157-66.

Efficiently closing an anterior open bite. Pellan P. Int J Orthod Milwaukee. 2008 Winter;19(4):44-5.

Long-term outcome in a patient with a dentoskeletal open-bite malocclusion treated without extraction. Celli D, Gasperoni E, Deli R. World J Orthod. 2007 Winter;8(4):344-56.

Correction of skeletal open bite with implant anchored molar/bicuspid intrusion. Sherwood K.Oral Maxillofac Surg Clin North Am. 2007 Aug;19(3):339-50, vi.

Anterior open bite correction by Le Fort I or bilateral sagittal split osteotomy. Reyneke JP, Ferretti C. Oral Maxillofac Surg Clin North Am. 2007 Aug;19(3):321-38, v.

Dentoalveolar open bite treatment with spur appliances. Meyer-Marcotty P, Hartmann J, Stellzig-Eisenhauer A.

J Orofac Orthop. 2007 Nov;68(6):510-21.

Treatment of severe anterior open bite with skeletal anchorage in adults: comparison with orthognathic surgery outcomes. Kuroda S, Sakai Y, Tamamura N, Deguchi T, Takano-Yamamoto T. Am J Orthod Dentofacial Orthop. 2007 Nov;132(5):599-605.

Protocol for the treatment of anterior open bite patients: an evaluation. Saldarriaga JR. World J Orthod. 2007 Fall;8(3):285-99.

Nonextraction and nonsurgical treatment of an adult with skeletal Class II open bite with severe retrognathic mandible and temporomandibular disorders. Kondo E. World J Orthod. 2007 Fall;8(3):261-76.

Early tooth extraction in the treatment of anterior open bite in hyperdivergent patients. de Figueiredo MA, Siqueira DF, Bommarito S, Sannomiya EK, White LW. World J Orthod. 2007 Fall;8(3):249-60.

Treating anterior open bite. Ren Y. Evid Based Dent. 2007;8(3):83.

Long-term Stability of Extraction Therapy in Anterior Open Bite. A Case Report. Muntean R, Komposch G, Steegmayer-Gilde G. J Orofac Orthop. 2007 Sep;68(5):413-22.

[Etiological aspects of anterior open bite]. Stojanović L. Med Pregl. 2007 Mar-Apr;60(3-4):151-5.

Surgical correction of a Class II skeletal malocclusion associated with anterior open bite and temporomandibular joint pain. Mendes Miguel JA, Cal-Neto JP, da Silveira HM. Am J Orthod Dentofacial Orthop. 2007 Sep;132(3):400-7.

Treatment and posttreatment effects of quad-helix/crib therapy of dentoskeletal open bite. Cozza P, Mucedero M, Baccetti T, Franchi L. Angle Orthod. 2007 Jul;77(4):640-5.

Posterior impaction with orthodontic miniscrews for openbite closure and improvement of facial profile. Kravitz ND, Kusnoto B. World J Orthod. 2007 Summer;8(2):157-66.

Stability following combined orthodontic-surgical treatment for skeletal anterior open bite - a cephalometric 15-year follow-up study. Ding Y, Xu TM, Lohrmann B, Gellrich NC, Schwestka-Polly R. J Orofac Orthop. 2007 May;68(3):245-56.

Anterior open bite and overjet treated with camouflage therapy. Denny JM, Weiskircher MA, Dorminey JC.

Am J Orthod Dentofacial Orthop. 2007 May;131(5):670-8.

Orthodontic and orthopaedic treatment for anterior open bite in children. Lentini-Oliveira D, Carvalho FR, Qingsong Y, Junjie L, Saconato H, Machado MA, Prado LB, Prado GF. Cochrane Database Syst Rev. 2007 Apr 18;(2):CD005515.

Anterior open bite with temporomandibular disorder treated with titanium screw anchorage: evaluation of morphological and functional improvement. Kuroda S, Sugawara Y, Tamamura N, Takano-Yamamoto T.

Am J Orthod Dentofacial Orthop. 2007 Apr;131(4):550-60.

Long-term skeletal stability after surgical correction in Class III open-bite patients: a retrospective study on 40 patients treated with mono- or bimaxillary surgery. Iannetti G, Fadda MT, Marianetti TM, Terenzi V, Cassoni A.

J Craniofac Surg. 2007 Mar;18(2):350-4.

A new approach in the treatment of skeletal open bite: vertically activated bite block. Arat ZM, Sezer FE, Arslan AD. World J Orthod. 2006 Winter;7(4):345-56.

Early treatment of skeletal open-bite malocclusion. Ren Y. Evid Based Dent. 2006;7(4):103.

Long-term stability of an anterior open-bite malocclusion treated in the mixed dentition: a case report.

de Almeida MR, de Almeida RR, Conti AC, Navarro Rde L, Correa Gde O, de Oliveira CA, Oltramari PV.

Anterior open bite treated with a palatal crib and high-pull chin cup therapy. A prospective randomized study.

Torres F, Almeida RR, de Almeida MR, Almeida-Pedrin RR, Pedrin F, Henriques JF. Eur J Orthod. 2006 Dec;28(6):610-7.

Dynamic MRI evaluation of tongue posture and deglutitive movements in a surgically corrected open bite.

Karacay S, Akin E, Ortakoglu K, Bengi AO. Angle Orthod. 2006 Nov;76(6):1057-65.

Microscrew anchorage in skeletal anterior open-bite treatment. Xun C, Zeng X, Wang X. Angle Orthod. 2007 Jan;77(1):47-56.

Cephalometric evaluation of anterior open-bite nonextraction treatment, using multiloop edgewise archwire therapy.

Endo T, Kojima K, Kobayashi Y, Shimooka S. Odontology. 2006 Sep;94(1):51-8.

Nonextraction treatment of an open bite with microscrew implant anchorage. Park HS, Kwon OW, Sung JH.

Am J Orthod Dentofacial Orthop. 2006 Sep;130(3):391-402.

A modified rapid palatal expander for correction of anterior open bite and posterior crossbite. Anhoury P.

J Clin Orthod. 2006 Aug;40(8):501.

Severe anterior open-bite malocclusion. Cal-Neto JP, Quintão CC, de Menezes LM, Almeida MA.

Angle Orthod. 2006 Jul;76(4):728-33.

Directional force treatment for an adult with Class III malocclusion and open bite. Lima CE, Lima MT.

Am J Orthod Dentofacial Orthop. 2006 Jun;129(6):817-24.

Stability of anterior open-bite extraction and nonextraction treatment in the permanent dentition. Janson G, Valarelli FP, Beltrão RT, de Freitas MR, Henriques JF. Am J Orthod Dentofacial Orthop. 2006 Jun;129(6):768-74.

Treatment effects of a modified quad-helix in patients with dentoskeletal open bites. Cozza P, Baccetti T, Franchi L, McNamara JA Jr. Am J Orthod Dentofacial Orthop. 2006 Jun;129(6):734-9.

Correction of anterior open bite in a case of achondroplasia. Karpagam S, Rabin K, George M, Santhosh K. Indian J Dent Res. 2005 Oct-Dec;16(4):159-66.

A retrospective and prospective view of orofacial myology. Mason RM. Int J Orofacial Myology. 2005 Nov;31:5-14.

Nonsurgical correction of an adult skeletal class III and open-bite malocclusion. Hamamci N, Başaran G, Sahin S.

Angle Orthod. 2006 May;76(3):527-32.

New generation open-bite treatment with zygomatic anchorage. Erverdi N, Usumez S, Solak A. Angle Orthod. 2006 May;76(3):519-26.

Initial effects of the tongue crib on tongue movements during deglutition: a Cine-Magnetic resonance imaging study. Sayin MO, Akin E, Karaçay S, Bulakbaşi N. Angle Orthod. 2006 May;76(3):400-5. Erratum in: Angle Orthod. 2006 Jul;76(4):iii.

A prospective study of the treatment effects of a removable appliance with palatal crib combined with high-pull chincup therapy in anterior open-bite patients. Pedrin F, Almeida MR, Almeida RR, Almeida-Pedrin RR, Torres F.

Am J Orthod Dentofacial Orthop. 2006 Mar;129(3):418-23.

Treatment of post-traumatic open bite by radiofrequency. Choi SS, Rotaru H, Kim SG. Br J Oral Maxillofac Surg. 2007 Jun;45(4):311-3.

Modified maxillary protraction headgear for the correction of class III skeletal malocclusion with anterior open bite.

Qazi HS, Amjad AT. J Coll Physicians Surg Pak. 2005 Dec;15(12):823-5.

[Anterior open bite: a formula for the differential diagnosis]. Alimere HC, Thomazinho A, de Felício CM.

Pro Fono. 2005 Apr-Dec;17(3):367-74. Portuguese.

Early orthodontic treatment of skeletal open-bite malocclusion: a systematic review. Cozza P, Mucedero M, Baccetti T, Franchi L. Angle Orthod. 2005 Sep;75(5):707-13. Review.

Preventive and interceptive orthodontic treatment needs of an inner-city group of 6- and 9-year-old Canadian children. Karaiskos N, Wiltshire WA, Odlum O, Brothwell D, Hassard TH. J Can Dent Assoc. 2005 Oct;71(9):649.

Prevalence and severity of malocclusion in adolescent Kuwaitis. Behbehani F, Artun J, Al-Jame B, Kerosuo H.

Med Princ Pract. 2005 Nov-Dec;14(6):390-5.

Equilibration of a progressive anterior open occlusal relationship: a clinical report. Solow RA.

Cranio. 2005 Jul;23(3):229-38.

Variations of the gonial angle in vertical surgical reduction of the maxillary-mandibular complex. Claudio R, Claudio U, Alessandro A, Massimiliano T, Angelo M. J Craniofac Surg. 2005 Jul;16(4):716-9.

Orthopedic approach in the treatment of a skeletal class II division 1 malocclusion with an anterior open bite.

Al-Sulaita N, White GE. J Clin Pediatr Dent. 2005 Spring;29(3):205-10.

An adult case of skeletal open bite with a large lower anterior facial height. Tanaka E, Iwabe T, Kawai N, Nishi M, Dalla-Bona D, Hasegawa T, Tanne K. Angle Orthod. 2005 May;75(3):465-71.

[Effect of the early intervention of oral habits on the development of dental occlusion]. Bertoldi PM, Felfício CM, Matsumoto MA. Pro Fono. 2005 Jan-Apr;17(1):37-44.

Nonsurgical treatment of adult open bite using edgewise appliance combined with high-pull headgear and class III elastics. Saito I, Yamaki M, Hanada K. Angle Orthod. 2005 Mar;75(2):277-83.

Attractiveness ratings of anterior open bites and reverse overjets using the aesthetic component of the Index of Orthodontic Treatment Need. Abu Alhaija ES, Al-Khateeb SN. Eur J Orthod. 2005 Apr;27(2):134-9.

Anterior open bite and disappearing condyles. Miller DB. Funct Orthod. 2002 Spring;19(1):16-23.

Treatment of open bite with microscrew implant anchorage. Park HS, Kwon TG, Kwon OW. Am J Orthod Dentofacial Orthop. 2004 Nov;126(5):627-36.

Severe anterior open-bite case treated using titanium screw anchorage. Kuroda S, Katayama A, Takano-Yamamoto T. Angle Orthod. 2004 Aug;74(4):558-67.

Initial intrusion of the molars in the treatment of anterior open bite malocclusions in growing patients. Gurton AU, Akin E, Karacay S. Angle Orthod. 2004 Aug;74(4):454-64.

The use of skeletal anchorage in open bite treatment: a cephalometric evaluation. Erverdi N, Keles A, Nanda R.

Angle Orthod. 2004 Jun;74(3):381-90.

Prevalence of malocclusions in the early mixed dentition and orthodontic treatment need. Tausche E, Luck O, Harzer W. Eur J Orthod. 2004 Jun;26(3):237-44.

[Biomechanical study of open bite treatment with tip forward bend]. Hu M, Li H, Liu L, Wu H, Chen YP, Xu YZ.

Zhonghua Kou Qiang Yi Xue Za Zhi. 2004 May;39(3):233-5.

Interdisciplinary treatment including forced extrusion and reintrusion of a traumatized mandibular incisor for a patient with Class II Division 1 skeletal open bite. Arvystas MG, Chivian N. Am J Orthod Dentofacial Orthop. 2004 Feb;125(2):206-12.

Skeletal and dental effects during observation and treatment with a magnetic device. Meral O, Yüksel S. Angle Orthod. 2003 Dec;73(6):716-22.

Long-term stability of anterior open bite extraction treatment in the permanent dentition. de Freitas MR, Beltrão RT, Janson G, Henriques JF, Cançado RH. Am J Orthod Dentofacial Orthop. 2004 Jan;125(1):78-87.

Lip sucking and lip biting in the primary dentition: two cases treated with a morphological approach combined with lip exercises and habituation. Fukumitsu K, Ohno F, Ohno T. Int J Orofacial Myology. 2003 Nov;29:42-57.

Orthodontic findings in the deciduous and early mixed dentition--inferences for a preventive strategy. Stahl F, Grabowski R. J Orofac Orthop. 2003 Nov;64(6):401-16. English, German.

An adolescent case of anterior open bite with masticatory muscle dysfunction. Tanaka E, Iwabe T, Watanabe M, Kato M, Tanne K. Angle Orthod. 2003 Oct;73(5):608-13.

Stability of anterior open bite nonextraction treatment in the permanent dentition. Janson G, Valarelli FP, Henriques JF, de Freitas MR, Cançado RH. Am J Orthod Dentofacial Orthop. 2003 Sep;124(3):265-76; quiz 340.

The causes, diagnosis and treatment of anterior open bite. Burford D, Noar JH. Dent Update. 2003 Jun;30(5):235-41.

Indication for and frequency of early orthodontic therapy or interceptive measures. Schopf P. J Orofac Orthop. 2003 May;64(3):186-200.

Dentofacial anomalies related to the digit sucking habit. daCosta OO, Orenuga OO. Afr J Med Med Sci. 2002 Sep;31(3):239-42.

The pattern of malocclusion among orthodontic patients seen in Dental Centre, University College Hospital, Ibadan, Nigeria. Onyeaso CO, Aderinokun GA, Arowojolu MO. Afr J Med Med Sci. 2002 Sep;31(3):207-11.

Severe anterior open bite malocclusion with multiple odontoma treated by C-lingual retractor and horseshoe mechanics. Kim S, Park Y, Chung K. Angle Orthod. 2003 Apr;73(2):206-12.

Does an anterior open bite in the early mixed dentition cause you to consider any form of orthodontic treatment?. Klocke A. Am J Orthod Dentofacial Orthop. 2003 Mar;123(3):13A. No abstract available.

Use of a tip-edge stage-1 wire to enhance vertical control during straight wire treatment: two case reports. Taylor H. Angle Orthod. 2003 Feb;73(1):93-9.

Indications and procedures for segmental dentoalveolar osteotomy: a review of 13 patients. Yokoo S, Komori T, Watatani S, Shibuya Y, Komurasaki H, Tateishi C. Int J Adult Orthodon Orthognath Surg. 2002;17(4):254-63.

Treatment and posttreatment dentoalveolar changes following intrusion of mandibular molars with application of a skeletal anchorage system (SAS) for open bite correction. Sugawara J, Baik UB, Umemori M, Takahashi I, Nagasaka H, Kawamura H, Mitani H. Int J Adult Orthodon Orthognath Surg. 2002;17(4):243-53.

Occlusal interferences in orthodontic patients before and after treatment, and in subjects with minor orthodontic treatment need. Olsson M, Lindqvist B. Eur J Orthod. 2002 Dec;24(6):677-87.

Moulding of the generate to control open bite during mandibular distraction osteogenesis. Peltomäki T, Grayson BH, Vendittelli BL, Katzen T, McCarthy JG. Eur J Orthod. 2002 Dec;24(6):639-45.

Closing anterior open bites by intruding molars with titanium miniplate anchorage. Sherwood KH, Burch JG, Thompson WJ. Am J Orthod Dentofacial Orthop. 2002 Dec;122(6):593-600.

[Anterior open bite: surgically or orthodontically treated]. Zou B, Zeng X, Zeng Y. Zhonghua Kou Qiang Yi Xue Za Zhi. 2002 Mar;37(2):139-41.

Effects of vertical chincap therapy on the mandibular morphology in open-bite patients. Işcan HN, Dinçer M, Gültan A, Meral O, Taner-Sarisoy L. Am J Orthod Dentofacial Orthop. 2002 Nov;122(5):506-11.

Correcting an anterior open-bite side effect during distraction with spring forces. Yen SL, Gross J, Yamashita DD, Kim TH, McAndrews J, Shuler C, Reinisch J. Plast Reconstr Surg. 2002 Nov;110(6):1476-84.

Effect of varying the force direction on maxillary orthopedic protraction. Keles A, Tokmak EC, Erverdi N, Nanda R.

Angle Orthod. 2002 Oct;72(5):387-96.

Lingual extraction treatment of anterior open bite in an adult. Geron S, Chaushu S. J Clin Orthod. 2002 Aug;36(8):441-6.

Vertical changes following orthodontic extraction treatment in skeletal open bite subjects. Aras A. Eur J Orthod. 2002 Aug;24(4):407-16.

Bilateral open bite in dicygotic twins. A combined orthodontic-prosthetic approach. Radlanski RJ, Freesmeyer WB.

J Orofac Orthop. 2002 Jul;63(4):339-47.

An adult case of skeletal open bite with a severely narrowed maxillary dental arch. Takeuchi M, Tanaka E, Nonoyama D, Aoyama J, Tanne K. Angle Orthod. 2002 Aug;72(4):362-70.

Correction of severe vertical maxillary excess with anterior open bite and transverse maxillary deficiency.

Conley RS, Legan HL. Angle Orthod. 2002 Jun;72(3):265-74.

Effects of a modified acrylic bonded rapid maxillary expansion appliance and vertical chin cap on dentofacial structures. Basciftci FA, Karaman AI. Angle Orthod. 2002 Feb;72(1):61-71.

Treatment of a Class III anterior open bite malocclusion: a combined orthodontic and orthognathic surgical approach. Ong HB. Singapore Dent J. 2001 Jun;24(1):35-42.

Treatment of a Class II division 1 anterior open bite malocclusion. Ong HB. Singapore Dent J. 2001 Jun;24(1):29-34.

Closing a severe anterior open-bite in a young adult. Sim JM. J Gen Orthod. 2001 Fall;12(3):30-1.

Vector control in lower jaw distraction osteogenesis using an extra-oral multidirectional device. Hurmerinta K, Hukki J. J Craniomaxillofac Surg. 2001 Oct;29(5):263-70.

Skeletal and dento-alveolar stability after surgical-orthodontic treatment of anterior open bite: a retrospective study.

Swinnen K, Politis C, Willems G, De Bruyne I, Fieuws S, Heidbuchel K, van Erum R, Verdonck A, Carels C.

Eur J Orthod. 2001 Oct;23(5):547-57.

Treatment of a Class II deformity with skeletal open bite and lateroocclusion. Watted N, Wieber M, Reuther J.

Clin Orthod Res. 2001 Feb;4(1):50-9.

[Distraction osteogenesis with double internal devices combined with early frontal facial advancement for the correction of facial craniosynostosis. Report of clinical cases]. Arnaud E, Marchac D, Renier D. Ann Chir Plast Esthet. 2001 Aug;46(4):268-76.

The functional treatment of anterior-open bite: three case reports. Dinçer B, Hazar S. J Clin Pediatr Dent. 2001 Summer;25(4):275-86.

[A study on improving tongue functions of open-bite children at the mixed dentition period--modifications of a removable habit-breaker appliance and their sonographic analysis]. Saito M. Kokubyo Gakkai Zasshi. 2001 Jun;68(2):193-207.

Effect of orthognathic surgery on the temporomandibular joint in patients with anterior open bite. Aghabeigi B, Hiranaka D, Keith DA, Kelly JP, Crean SJ. Int J Adult Orthodon Orthognath Surg. 2001;16(2):153-60.

Severe dental open bite malocclusion with tongue reduction after orthodontic treatment. Hotokezaka H, Matsuo T, Nakagawa M, Mizuno A, Kobayashi K. Angle Orthod. 2001 Jun;71(3):228-36.

[Stability of orthodontic-maxillofacial surgical treatment of anterior open bite deformities]]. Hoppenreijs TJ, Freihofer HP, Stoelinga PJ, Tuinzing DB. Ned Tijdschr Tandheelkd. 2001 May;108(5):173-8.

Long-term dentofacial stability after bimaxillary surgery in skeletal Class III open bite patients. Moldez MA, Sugawara J, Umemori M, Mitani H, Kawamura H. Int J Adult Orthodon Orthognath Surg. 2000 Winter;15(4):309-19.

Anterior open-bite malocclusion: stability of maxillary repositioning using rigid internal fixation. Arpornmaeklong P, Heggie AA. Aust Orthod J. 2000 Jul;16(2):69-81.

Electropalatographic and cephalometric assessment of myofunctional therapy in open-bite subjects. Cayley AS, Tindall AP, Sampson WJ, Butcher AR. Aust Orthod J. 2000 Mar;16(1):23-33.

Stability of anterior open bite correction with MEAW. Huang GJ, Drangsholt M. Am J Orthod Dentofacial Orthop. 2001 Feb;119(2):14A.

Effects of spring-loaded posterior bite-block appliance on masticatory muscles. Akkaya S, Haydar S, Bilir E.

Am J Orthod Dentofacial Orthop. 2000 Aug;118(2):179-83.

Bimaxillary orthognathic surgery in a patient with long face: a case report. Ataoğlu H, Uçkan S, Karaman AI, Uyar Y. Int J Adult Orthodon Orthognath Surg. 1999;14(4):304-9.

Nonsurgical management of the anterior open bite: a review of the options. Beane RA Jr. Semin Orthod. 1999 Dec;5(4):275-83.

Long-term stability of surgical open-bite correction by Le Fort I osteotomy. Proffit WR, Bailey LJ, Phillips C, Turvey TA. Angle Orthod. 2000 Apr;70(2):112-7.

Nonsurgical and nonextraction treatment of skeletal Class III open bite: its long-term stability. Kondo E, Aoba TJ.

Am J Orthod Dentofacial Orthop. 2000 Mar;117(3):267-87.

Psychologic implications of surgical-orthodontic treatment in patients with anterior open bite. Hoppenreijs TJ, Hakman EC, van't Hof MA, Stoelinga PJ, Tuinzing DB, Freihofer HP. Int J Adult Orthodon Orthognath Surg. 1999;14(2):101-12.

The effects of a modified protraction headgear on maxilla. Alcan T, Keles A, Erverdi N. Am J Orthod Dentofacial Orthop. 2000 Jan;117(1):27-38.

Cephalometric evaluation of open bite treatment with NiTi arch wires and anterior elastics. Küçükkeleş N, Acar A, Demirkaya AA, Evrenol B, Enacar A. Am J Orthod Dentofacial Orthop. 1999 Nov;116(5):555-62.

Open bite, dental alveolar protrusion, class I malocclusion: A successful treatment result. Alexander CD.

Am J Orthod Dentofacial Orthop. 1999 Nov;116(5):494-500.

Evidence of correction of open bite malocclusion using active vertical corrector treatment. Bazzucchi A, Hans MG, Nelson S, Powers M, Parker S. Semin Orthod. 1999 Jun;5(2):110-20.

Long-term stability of treatment results after upper jaw segmented osteotomy according to Schuchardt for correction of anterior open bite. Ermel T, Hoffmann J, Alfter G, Göz G. J Orofac Orthop. 1999;60(4):236-45.

Habitual snoring, OSA and craniofacial modification. Orthodontic clinical and diagnostic aspects in a case control study. Caprioglio A, Zucconi M, Calori G, Troiani V. Minerva Stomatol. 1999 Apr;48(4):125-37.

Tongue muscle activity after orthodontic treatment of anterior open bite: a case report. Yashiro K, Takada K.

Am J Orthod Dentofacial Orthop. 1999 Jun;115(6):660-6.

Nonsurgical correction of a skeletal Class II, Division 1, malocclusion with bilateral crossbite and anterior open bite.

Sabri R. Am J Orthod Dentofacial Orthop. 1998 Aug;114(2):189-94.

Influence of orthodontic treatment in the primary dentition upon development of the dentition and craniofacial growth. Mauck C, Tränkmann J. J Orofac Orthop. 1998;59(4):229-36.

[An experimental study of a new bidirectional distraction appliance]. Lucas R, Gounot N, Cresseaux P, Breton P, Freidel M, Ferez C,

Roger T, Genevois JP. Rev Stomatol Chir Maxillofac. 1998 Jul;99 Suppl 1:72-5.

A clinical technique for the management of a Class II skeletal relationship with an anterior open bite as a result of long face syndrome in the adult patient. Bixby GK. Funct Orthod. 1998 Jan-Feb;15(1):22-3, 26-7.

Extraction treatment of a Class II, Division 1 malocclusion with anterior open bite with headgear and vertical elastics. Gehring D, Freeseman M, Frazier M, Southard K. Am J Orthod Dentofacial Orthop. 1998 Apr;113(4):431-6.

Effect of presurgical incisor extrusion on stability of anterior open bite malocclusion treated with orthognathic surgery. Lo FM, Shapiro PA. Int J Adult Orthodon Orthognath Surg. 1998;13(1):23-34.

Stability of transverse maxillary dental arch dimensions following orthodontic-surgical correction of anterior open bites. Hoppenreijs TJ, van der Linden FP, Freihofer HP, Stoelinga PJ, Tuinzing DB, Jacobs BT, van 't Hof MA.

Int J Adult Orthodon Orthognath Surg. 1998;13(1):7-22.

The nature of arch width difference and palatal depth of the anterior open bite. Hsu BS. Am J Orthod Dentofacial Orthop. 1998 Mar;113(3):344-50.

Cephalometric evaluation of dento-skeletal changes during treatment with the Bionator type 1. Carels C, Reychler A, van der Linden FP. J Oral Rehabil. 1997 Nov;24(11):841-8.

Comparison of the effects of passive posterior bite-blocks with different construction bites on the craniofacial and dentoalveolar structures. Iscan HN, Sarisoy L. Am J Orthod Dentofacial Orthop. 1997 Aug;112(2):171-8.

Skeletal and dento-alveolar stability of Le Fort I intrusion osteotomies and bimaxillary osteotomies in anterior open bite deformities. A retrospective three-centre study. Hoppenreijs TJ, Freihofer HP, Stoelinga PJ, Tuinzing DB, van't Hof MA, van der Linden FP, Nottet SJ. Int J Oral Maxillofac Surg. 1997 Jun;26(3):161-75.

Open bite: a review of etiology and management. Ngan P, Fields HW. Pediatr Dent. 1997 Mar-Apr;19(2):91-8.

A diagnostic index of vertical problems for Class III malocclusions. Miyajima K, McNamara JA Jr, Murata S.

Int J Adult Orthodon Orthognath Surg. 1997;12(3):189-95.

The stability of the use of bilateral sagittal split osteotomy in the closure of anterior open bite. Oliveira JA, Bloomquist DS. Int J Adult Orthodon Orthognath Surg. 1997;12(2):101-8.

The effectiveness of orofacial myofunctional therapy in improving dental occlusion. Benkert KK.

Int J Orofacial Myology. 1997;23:35-46.

Outcome prediction of the anterior open bite. Comparison of computer and clinician analysis of cephalograms.

McSherry PF, Richardson A, Turner J. J Orofac Orthop. 1997;58(5):262-9.

Bonded magnets used in the treatment of anterior open bite. Reply to Dr. Dellinger (previously printed in the September 1996 issue) Noar JH. Am J Orthod Dentofacial Orthop. 1997 Jan;111(1):16A-17A.

Treatment of an adult with a severe anterior open bite and mutilated malocclusion without orthognathic surgery.

Smith GA. Am J Orthod Dentofacial Orthop. 1996 Dec;110(6):682-7.

Active vertical corrector treatment--long-term follow-up of anterior open bite treated by the intrusion of posterior teeth. Dellinger EL, Dellinger EL. Am J Orthod Dentofacial Orthop. 1996 Aug;110(2):145-54.

An American Board of Orthodontics case report: the orthodontic-surgical correction of a Class II malocclusion with anterior open bite. Glenn G. Am J Orthod Dentofacial Orthop. 1996 Jul;110(1):81-7.

The performance of bonded magnets used in the treatment of anterior open bite. Noar JH, Shell N, Hunt NP.

Am J Orthod Dentofacial Orthop. 1996 May;109(5):549-56; discussion 557.

The physical properties and behavior of magnets used in the treatment of anterior open bite. Noar JH, Shell N, Hunt NP. Am J Orthod Dentofacial Orthop. 1996 Apr;109(4):437-44.

Comparison of computed tomography imaging before and after functional treatment of bilateral condylar fractures in adults. Choi BH. Int J Oral Maxillofac Surg. 1996 Feb;25(1):30-3.

Functional characteristics of patients with anterior open bite before and after surgical correction. Ellis E 3rd, Throckmorton G, Sinn DP. Int J Adult Orthodon Orthognath Surg. 1996;11(3):211-23.

An etiology and treatment of anterior open bite. McSherry PF. J Ir Dent Assoc. 1996;42(2):20-6.

Occlusal and functional conditions after surgical correction of anterior open bite deformities. Hoppenreijs TJ, van der Linden FP, Freihofer HP, van 't Hof MA, Tuinzing DB, Voorsmit RA, Stoelinga PJ. Int J Adult Orthodon Orthognath Surg. 1996;11(1):29-39.

Nonsurgical treatment of open bite in nongrowing patients. Sarver DM, Weissman SM. Am J Orthod Dentofacial Orthop. 1995 Dec;108(6):651-9.

Oral myiasis: report of two cases. al-Ismaily M, Scully C. Int J Paediatr Dent. 1995 Sep;5(3):177-9.

Treatment of the craniofacial complications of Beckwith-Wiedemann syndrome. Menard RM, Delaire J, Schendel SA. Plast Reconstr Surg. 1995 Jul;96(1):27-33.

The effects of Frankel's function regulator (FR-4) therapy on the treatment of Angle Class I skeletal anterior open bite malocclusion. Erbay E, Uğur T, Ulgen M. Am J Orthod Dentofacial Orthop. 1995 Jul;108(1):9-21.

The anterior open bite problem (infraclusion). Champagne M. J Gen Orthod. 1995 Jun;6(2):5-10. Review.

The assessment and treatment of anterior open bite. Ferguson JW. Dent Update. 1995 May;22(4):163-8. Review.

Partial glossectomy for the treatment of anterior open bite. A case report. Ball JV, Horrocks EN. Br J Orthod. 1995 May;22(2):185-9.

The use of implants for orthodontic correction of an open bite. Prosterman B, Prosterman L, Fisher R, Gornitsky M.

Am J Orthod Dentofacial Orthop. 1995 Mar;107(3):245-50.

A combined orthodontic and orthognathic surgery approach to the treatment of extreme anterior open bite in an adult. Dearing SG. N Z Dent J. 1994 Dec;90(402):143-7.

Case report--anterior open bite as a complication of splint therapy. Todd MA, Freer TJ. Aust Orthod J. 1994 Oct;13(3):164-7.

Vertical elastics for correction of anterior open bite. Rinchuse DJ. J Clin Orthod. 1994 May;28(5):284.

Case report: nonsurgical treatment of an adult with severe anterior open bite. Goto S, Boyd RL, Iizuka T. Angle Orthod. 1994;64(4):311-8.

Treating orofacial dyskinesia with functional physiotherapy in the case of frontal open bite. Daglio SD, Schwitzer R, Wüthrich J, Kallivroussis G. Int J Orofacial Myology. 1993 Nov;19:11-4.

Cephalometric evaluation of maxillary retrognathism cases treated with FR-3 appliance. Biren S, Erverdi N.

J Marmara Univ Dent Fac. 1993 Sep;1(4):354-60.

Anterior open bite malocclusion: a follow-up study of orthodontic treatment effects. Katsaros C, Berg R.

Eur J Orthod. 1993 Aug;15(4):273-80.

Imperative early treatment of anterior open bite. Chase WR. Gen Dent. 1993 Jul-Aug;41(4):307-9. Review.

Occlusal plane rotation: aesthetic enhancement in mandibular micrognathia. Rosen HM. Plast Reconstr Surg. 1993 Jun;91(7):1231-40; discussion 1241-4.

Treatment of anterior open bite with tongue thrust and associated temporo-mandibular joint symptoms. Lee BW.

Aust Orthod J. 1993 Mar;12(4):246-9. No abstract available.

The effect of treatment of skeletal open bite with two types of bite-blocks. Kuster R, Ingervall B. Eur J Orthod. 1992 Dec;14(6):489-99.

Functional regulator therapy in treatment of skeletal open-bite. Haydar B, Enacar A. J Nihon Univ Sch Dent. 1992 Dec;34(4):278-87.

[Anterior open bite]. Hoppenreijs TJ, van der Linden FP. Ned Tijdschr Tandheelkd. 1992 Nov;99(11):444-9. Dutch.

Stability of surgical correction of patients with Skeletal III and Skeletal II anterior open bite, with increased maxillary mandibular planes angle. McCance AM, Moss JP, James DR. Eur J Orthod. 1992 Jun;14(3):198-206.

Mandibular autorotation in orthognathic surgery: a new method of locating the centre of mandibular rotation and determining its consequence in orthognathic surgery. Nattestad A, Vedtofte P. J Craniomaxillofac Surg. 1992 May-Jun;20(4):163-70.

Skeletal and dento-alveolar changes as a result of headgear activator therapy related to different vertical growth patterns. Dermaut LR, van den Eynde F, de Pauw G. Eur J Orthod. 1992 Apr;14(2):140-6.

Cephalometric changes during treatment with the open bite bionator. Weinbach JR, Smith RJ. Am J Orthod Dentofacial Orthop. 1992 Apr;101(4):367-74.

Assessment of orthodontic treatment needs by teenagers in an Asian community in Singapore. Soh G, Lew KK.

Community Dent Health. 1992 Mar;9(1):57-62.

Patterns of incisor root resorption before and after orthodontic correction in cases with anterior open bites.

Harris EF, Butler ML. Am J Orthod Dentofacial Orthop. 1992 Feb;101(2):112-9.

The effects of the spring-loaded posterior bite-block on the maxillo-facial morphology. Işcan HN, Akkaya S, Koralp E. Eur J Orthod. 1992 Feb;14(1):54-60.

Case report SH. Combined surgical and orthodontic treatment of an anterior open bite. Twesme DA, Sarver DM, Matukas VJ. Angle Orthod. 1992 Spring;62(1):77-80. No abstract available.

Post-treatment effects of the Herbst appliance. A radiographic, clinical and biometric investigation. Hansen K.

Swed Dent J Suppl. 1992;88:1-49.

[Anterior open bite]. Champagne M. Inf Dent. 1991 Dec 5;73(42):3875-81. Review. French. No abstract available.

Advanced periodontal disease and development of anterior open bite. A case report. Zubery Y, Machtei EE.

Am J Dent. 1991 Dec;4(6):295-7.

Screw fixation after mandibular sagittal split osteotomy: an intra-oral approach. Shepherd JP, Dohvoma CN, Harradine NW. Br J Oral Maxillofac Surg. 1991 Oct;29(5):325-9.

The influence of tonsillar obstruction and tonsillectomy on facial growth and dental arch morphology. Hultcrantz E, Larson M, Hellquist R, Ahlquist-Rastad J, Svanholm H, Jakobsson OP. Int J Pediatr Otorhinolaryngol. 1991 Sep;22(2):125-34.

Surgical orthodontic treatment of anterior skeletal open bite using small plate internal fixation. One to five year follow-up. Haymond CS, Stoelinga PJ, Blijdorp PA, Leenen RJ, Merkens NM. Int J Oral Maxillofac Surg. 1991 Aug;20(4):223-7.

Temporalis and masseter muscle activity in patients with anterior open bite and craniomandibular disorders.

Bakke M, Michler L. Scand J Dent Res. 1991 Jun;99(3):219-28.

A ten-year follow-up case report following surgical correction of anterior open bite. Lew KK, Loh HS.

Aust Dent J. 1991 Apr;36(2):109-12.

[Vertical-sagittal "peninsular" osteotomy of the body of the mandible: a concept for forward displacement and anterior rotation of the mandible]. Höltje WJ, Scheuer HA. Fortschr Kieferorthop. 1991 Feb;52(1):34-9. German.

[Clinical experience in surgical-orthodontic treatment of patients with anterior skeletal open-bite]. Silvestri A, Spagnuolo A, Natali G. Mondo Ortod. 1991 Jan-Feb;16(1):35-49. Italian.

Anterior open bite treatment with magnets. Kiliaridis S, Egermark I, Thilander B. Eur J Orthod. 1990 Nov;12(4):447-57.

A longitudinal study on malocclusion in relation to signs and symptoms of cranio-mandibular disorders in children and adolescents. Egermark-Eriksson I, Carlsson GE, Magnusson T, Thilander B. Eur J Orthod. 1990 Nov;12(4):399-407.

An esthetic approach to vertical root extrusion in a patient with an anterior open bite: report of case. Hartwell GR, McDonnell CJ 3rd. J Am Dent Assoc. 1990 Oct;121(4):515-7.

[Modified Klammt apparatus for treatment of stomatognathic abnormalities in preschool children]. Piekarczyk B.

Czas Stomatol. 1990 Oct;43(10):623-8. Polish.

Combined orthodontic and restorative correction of severe anterior open bite. Cooke MS, Neesome PR.

Quintessence Int. 1990 Sep;21(9):729-36.

An American Board of Orthodontics case report. Treatment of an open bite malocclusion. Efstratiadis SS.

Am J Orthod Dentofacial Orthop. 1990 Aug;98(2):94-102.

Adult anterior open bite. Galletto L, Urbaniak J, Subtelny JD. Am J Orthod Dentofacial Orthop. 1990 Jun;97(6):522-6. No abstract available.

[Treatments of major skeletal anomalies in adults]. Krogstad O. Nor Tannlaegeforen Tid. 1990 Jun;100(9):396-403. Norwegian.

[Prevalence of malocclusions and demand for orthodontic treatment among students at a women's high school].

Kitai N, Takada K, Yasuda Y, Adachi S, Hirase E, Kitaguchi T, Sakuda M. Osaka Daigaku Shigaku Zasshi. 1990 Jun;35(1):321-7. Japanese.

[Anterior open bite. Concept, etiology, characteristics, classification and clinical cases]. da Silva Ursi WJ, de Almeida RR. RGO. 1990 May-Jun;38(3):211-4, 217-8. Review. Portuguese.

[The functional regulators (FR III, FR IV)]. Işiksal E, Seçkin O. Turk Ortodonti Derg. 1990 Apr;3(1):150-6. Turkish.

A review of the management of anterior open bite malocclusion. Lawry DM, Heggie AA, Crawford EC, Ruljancich MK. Aust Orthod J. 1990 Mar;11(3):147-60. Review.

Anterior open bite. Etiology and treatment. Rodrigues de Almeida R, Ursi WJ. Oral Health. 1990 Jan;80(1):27-31. No abstract available.

The surgical treatment of skeletal anterior open-bite deformities with rigid internal fixation in the mandible.

Reitzik M, Barer PG, Wainwright WM, Lim B. Am J Orthod Dentofacial Orthop. 1990 Jan;97(1):52-7.

[Case of skeletal open bite treated with orthognathic surgery, with special reference to morphological and functional analysis of the tongue]. Koh Y, Tsuchiya M, Adachi S, Yoshida K, Sakuda M. Nihon Kyosei Shika Gakkai Zasshi. 1989 Dec;48(6):623-34. Japanese.

Vertical and horizontal components of functional appliance therapy. Moore RN, Igel KA, Boice PA. Am J Orthod Dentofacial Orthop. 1989 Nov;96(5):433-43.

[Open bite: orthodontic prosthetic surgical treatment. Presentation of a case]. Casanova PR, Zaldivar ER, Hidalgo Hidalgo S. Rev Cubana Estomatol. 1989 Jul-Sep;26(3):181-90. Spanish.

An American Board of Orthodontics case report. Snyder DE. Am J Orthod Dentofacial Orthop. 1989 Jun;95(6):451-6.

[Case reports and discussion on anterior open bite]. Hwang CJ, Baik HS. Taehan Chikkwa Uisa Hyophoe Chi. 1989 May;27(5):477-89. Korean.

[Thumbsucking and malocclusion--presentation of a clinical case]. Estripeaut LE, Henriques JF, de Almeida RR.

Rev Odontol Univ Sao Paulo. 1989 Apr-Jun;3(2):371-6. Portuguese.

[The assessment of nasopharyngeal airway space]. Dechkunakorn S, Sawaengkit P. J Dent Assoc Thai. 1989 Mar-Apr;39(2):43-50. Thai.

[A pathological consideration of ankyloglossia and lingual myoplasty]. Lee SK, Kim YS, Lim CY. Taehan Chikkwa Uisa Hyophoe Chi. 1989 Mar;27(3):287-308. Korean.

Cephalometric and clinical diagnoses of open bite tendency. Dung DJ, Smith RJ. Am J Orthod Dentofacial Orthop. 1988 Dec;94(6):484-90.

[A case report of anterior open bite with anterior crowding]. Ryu YK, Hwang HS, Kim YJ. Taehan Chikkwa Uisa Hyophoe Chi. 1988 Oct;26(10):935-44. Korean. No abstract available.

Adenotonsillectomy in children: indications and contraindications. Kavanagh KT, Beckford NS. South Med J. 1988 Apr;81(4):507-14.

Patterns of vertical growth in the face. Nanda SK. Am J Orthod Dentofacial Orthop. 1988 Feb;93(2):103-16.

Surgical treatment of the open bite deformity. Surgical correction of combined mandibular prognathism and open bite by oblique sliding osteotomy of the mandibular rami. Kahnberg KE, Widmark G. Int J Oral Maxillofac Surg. 1988 Feb;17(1):45-8.

Surgical superior maxillary repositioning and mandibular arch expansion for anterior open bite and internal derangement. Williamson EH. Facial Orthop Temporomandibular Arthrol. 1987 Oct;4(10):3-6. No abstract available.

Postero-lateral expansion osteotomy of maxilla. A case report. Merville LC, Princ G. J Craniomaxillofac Surg. 1987 Feb;15(1):20-3.

An American Board of Orthodontics case report. Pair DE. Am J Orthod Dentofacial Orthop. 1987 Feb;91(2):137-42.

Steroid-induced anterior open bite. Case report. Acton CH. Aust Dent J. 1986 Dec;31(6):455-8. No abstract available.

Facial morphology and obstructive sleep apnea. Lowe AA, Santamaria JD, Fleetham JA, Price C. Am J Orthod Dentofacial Orthop. 1986 Dec;90(6):484-91.

Relapse following surgical treatment of anterior open bite. Lansley CV, Stirrups DR, Moos KF. Br J Oral Maxillofac Surg. 1986 Dec;24(6):391-404.

Mandibular orthopedic change and closure of anterior open bite following reduction of disk dislocation.

Williamson EH. Facial Orthop Temporomandibular Arthrol. 1986 Jul;3(7):3-7. No abstract available.

A clinical assessment of the Active Vertical Corrector--a nonsurgical alternative for skeletal open bite treatment.

Dellinger EL. Am J Orthod. 1986 May;89(5):428-36.

A non-surgical approach to an anterior open bite: report of a case. Goldfogel M, Noonan JE Jr. Gerodontics. 1986 Feb;2(1):39-42. No abstract available.

Treatment of temporomandibular dysfunction and anterior open bite. Williamson EH.

Facial Orthop Temporomandibular Arthrol. 1985 Oct;2(10):4-7. No abstract available.

The influence of perennial allergic rhinitis on facial type and a pilot study of the effect of allergy management on facial growth patterns. Sassouni V, Friday GA, Shnorhokian H, Beery QC, Zullo TG, Miller DL, Murphey SM, Landay RA. Ann Allergy. 1985 Jun;54(6):493-7.

Orthodontic treatment and tongue surgery in a class III open-bite malocclusion. A case report. Ruff RM.

Angle Orthod. 1985 Apr;55(2):155-66.

Köle's osteotomy, a follow-up study. Kloosterman J. J Maxillofac Surg. 1985 Apr;13(2):59-63.

Anterior open-bite malocclusion: a longitudinal 10-year postretention evaluation of orthodontically treated patients.

Lopez-Gavito G, Wallen TR, Little RM, Joondeph DR. Am J Orthod. 1985 Mar;87(3):175-86.

Components of adult Class II open-bite malocclusion. Ellis E 3rd, McNamara JA Jr, Lawrence TM. J Oral Maxillofac Surg. 1985 Feb;43(2):92-105.

[Anterior open bite: the role of the infra-alveolae in its diagnosis and treatment]. Scheffer P, Verdier M, Hejazi H, Lerondeau JC, Laborie B. Rev Stomatol Chir Maxillofac. 1985;86(2):87-9. French.

Components of adult Class III open-bite malocclusion. Ellis E 3rd, McNamara JA Jr. Am J Orthod. 1984 Oct;86(4):277-90.

[Surgical approach of a vertical problem: the long face syndrome]. Casteigt J, Dereudre B.

Rev Stomatol Chir Maxillofac. 1984;85(2):83-93. French.

[Vertical maxillo-mandibular dysmorphias due to excessive growth. Terminology, diagnosis and treatment].

Merville LC, Diner PA. Rev Stomatol Chir Maxillofac. 1984;85(1):12-22. French.

[Postoperative changes of mandible and anterior teeth in orthognathic surgery for the correction of skeletal Class III open bite cases]. Sasakura H, Uchida H, Hirose H, Yamazaki O, Hanada K,

Ueda K, Nakajima T. Nihon Kyosei Shika Gakkai Zasshi. 1982 Jun;41(2):369-80. Japanese. No abstract available.

The surgical correction of vertical maxillary excess (long face syndrome). Angelillo JC, Dolan EA.

Ann Plast Surg. 1982 Jan;8(1):64-70.

Temporomandibular joint ankylosis--experience with a case of twenty years' duration. Minami RT.

Ann Plast Surg. 1981 Sep;7(3):228-32.

Anterior open bite. Orthodontic aspects--part 1. Cooke MS. Dent Update. 1980 Nov-Dec;7(6):475-6, 478-81. No abstract available.

The bite plate--an adjunct in periodontic and orthodontic therapy. Kessler M. J Periodontol. 1980 Mar;51(3):123-35. Review.

Diagnosis and treatment principles for anterior open bite malocclusions. Storey AT. Ont Dent. 1980 Mar;57(3):12-8. No abstract available.

[Anterior vertical open-bite between maxilla and mandible. Secondary surgical reduction]. Merville L. Orthod Fr. 1980;51:425-40. French. No abstract available.

Closed vertical subcondylar osteotomy (CVSO) of the mandible. A most versatile procedure. Tarsitano JJ, Gossman JR Jr. Int J Oral Surg. 1979 Dec;8(6):478-86.

Spontaneous regression of anterior open bite following treatment of macroglossia. Maisels DO, Knowles CC.

Br J Plast Surg. 1979 Oct;32(4):309-14.

[Relapse after mandibular advancement ina case of class II malocclusion with anterior open bite: a possible solution]. Litt R. Orthod Fr. 1979;50:447-59. French. No abstract available.

Digital sucking and tongue thrusting in children. Gellin ME. Dent Clin North Am. 1978 Oct;22(4):603-19.

Surgical correction of anterior open bite. Hayward JR. Int J Oral Surg. 1978 Aug;7(4):286-8. No abstract available.

Dental health in a group of Swedish 8-year-olds followed since the age of 3. Holm AK. Community Dent Oral Epidemiol. 1978 Mar;6(2):71-7.

Surgical-orthodontic correction of vertical maxillary excess. Fish LC, Wolford LM, Epker BN.

Am J Orthod. 1978 Mar;73(3):241-57.

Combined surgical and orthodontic management of anterior open bite using corticotomy. Generson RM, Porter JM, Zell A, Stratigos GT. J Oral Surg. 1978 Mar;36(3):216-9.

[The improvement of anterior open-bite with tongue thrusting in the early phase--a case report (author's transl)].

Hozaki T, Itooka T. Josai Shika Daigaku Kiyo. 1978;7(1):211-8. Japanese. No abstract available.

Treatment of anterior skeletal open-bite deformity. Arvystas MG. Am J Orthod. 1977 Aug;72(2):147-64.

Vertical proportions: a guide for prognosis and treatment in anterior open-bite. Nahoum HI. Am J Orthod. 1977 Aug;72(2):128-46.

A simple technique for the treatment of anterior open-bite due to a tongue thrust habit at an early age. Vojdani A.

Pa Dent J (Harrisb). 1977 May;44(3):14-5. No abstract available.

Surgical-orthodontic correction of open-bite deformity. Epker BN, Fish L. Am J Orthod. 1977 Mar;71(3):278-99.

Sagittal osteotomy of the mandibular horizontal ramus for correction of apertognathia: report of case. Kempf KK.

J Oral Surg. 1977 Mar;35(3):222-5.

Correction of anterior open bite deformity: a study of tongue function, speech changes, and stability. Turvey TA, Journot V, Epker BN. J Maxillofac Surg. 1976 Jun;4(2):93-101.

[Orthodontic, orthopedic and surgical treatment of anterior open bite]. Duchateaux C. Rev Orthop Dento Faciale. 1975 Jul;9(3):277-92. French. No abstract available.

Anterior open-bite: a cephalometric analysis and suggested treatment procedures. Nahoum HI.

Am J Orthod. 1975 May;67(5):523-21. No abstract available.

Overbite depth indicator with particular reference to anterior open-bite. Kim YH. Am J Orthod. 1974 Jun;65(6):586-611. No abstract available.

The treatment of anterior open bite with removable appliances. Heckmann U. Trans Eur Orthod Soc. 1974:173-80. No abstract available.

[Lower Schwarz plate with lingual obturator in the treatment of open bite in anterior segment]. Przylipiak S.

Czas Stomatol. 1973 Feb;26(2):177-83. Polish. No abstract available.

Tongue-thrust therapy and anterior dental open-bite. A review of new facial growth data. Speidel TM, Isaacson RJ, Worms FW. Am J Orthod. 1972 Sep;62(3):287-95. Review. No abstract available.

Surgical correction of anterior open bite: a case report. Anand SC. J Indian Dent Assoc. 1972 Jan;44(1):15-8. No abstract available.

Correction of skeletal type of anterior open bite. Bell WH. J Oral Surg. 1971 Oct;29(10):706-14. No abstract available.

Facial growth and the prognosis for anterior open-bite. A longitudinal study. Richardson A. Trans Eur Orthod Soc. 1971:149-57. No abstract available.

[Anterior open-bite]. Reychler A, Proost J. Acta Stomatol Belg. 1971;68(1):117-23. Dutch. No abstract available.

[Surgical treatment of anterior open bite]. Zemla J. Czas Stomatol. 1970 May;23(5):517-23. Polish. No abstract available.

Surgical correction of anterior open bite by sliding osteotomy. Bartlett GC. J N C Dent Soc. 1970 Jan;53(1):23-6. No abstract available.

Anterior open bite deformities and their correction by local osteotomy and bone graft. James PL. Trans Int Conf Oral Surg. 1970:24-31. No abstract available.

The early treatment of anterior open bite. Miller H. Int J Orthod. 1969 Mar;7(1):5-14. No abstract available.

Treatment of anterior open bite malocclusions. Rein B. Int J Orthod. 1969 Mar;7(1):27-34. No abstract available.

Generalized muscular weakness with severe anterior open-bite. A case report. Proffit WR, Gamble JW, Christiansen RL. Am J Orthod. 1968 Feb;54(2):104-10. No abstract available.

Maxillary and mandibular subapical osteotomies for the correction of anterior open-bite. Taylor RG, Mills PB, Brenner LD. Oral Surg Oral Med Oral Pathol. 1967 Feb;23(2):141-7. No abstract available.

A cephalometric investigation of skeletal factors in anterior open bite and deep overbite. Richardson A.

Rep Congr Eur Orthod Soc. 1967:159-71. No abstract available.

Anterior open-bite or retrognathia corrected by a vertical sliding osteotomy of the ramus, with or without bone graft: an improved technique. Preliminary report of two cases. CHRISTENSEN RW. Oral Surg Oral Med Oral Pathol. 1960 Dec;13:1409-22. No abstract available.

List of Thumb Suck Books Found on Google:

Some Love
Thumbs Up, Brown Bear
Open the Thumb Sucking Child
David Decides About Thumb Sucking
Why the Long Face: A Book About Thumb Sucking
My Thumb and I
Funny Teeth and Bunny Ears
Little Thumb
Mia's Thumb
Thumbuddy to Love Ballerina Sue
Jake's Best Thumb
Pacifiers Anonymous
My Thumb
Harold's Hideaway Thumb
Thumbsucker
The Quitting Deal
I'm Not a Vampire, I Just Suck My Thumb
It's No Fun Sucking Your Thumb
Goodbye, Thumbsucking
Bye-bye, Thumbsucking
How to Stop Thumb Sucking and Other Oral Habits: Practical Solutions for Home and Therapy
Danny and His Thumb
Donald Says Thumbs
The Wee Kitten Who Sucked Her Thumb
El Dedito de Kiki
Helping the Thumbsucking Child: A Practical Guide for Parents.

INDEX

Made in the USA
Monee, IL
08 November 2026

67384888R00152